Parish Nursing

Verna Benner Carson & Harold G. Koenig

Parish Nursing
Stories of Service and Care

REVISED EDITION

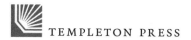
TEMPLETON PRESS

Templeton Press
300 Conshohocken State Road, Suite 550
West Conshohocken, PA 19428
www.templetonpress.org

Designed and typeset by Kachergis Book Design

Library of Congress Cataloging-in-Publication Data
Carson, Verna Benner.
Parish nursing : stories of service and care / Verna Benner Carson,
Harold G. Koenig. — Rev. ed.
p. ; cm.
Includes bibliographical references and index.
ISBN-13: 978-1-59947-348-2 (pbk. : alk. paper)
ISBN-10: 1-59947-348-8 (pbk. : alk. paper)   1. Parish nursing—United
States.   2. Parish nursing—United States—Anecdotes.   3. Pastoral
medicine—United States.   I. Koenig, Harold G. (Harold George), 1951–
II. Title.
[DNLM: 1. Nursing—United States.   2. Spirituality—United States.
3. Community Health Nursing—United States.   4. Religion and
Medicine—United States. WY 145]
RT120.P37C374 2011
610.73′43—dc22
2010035390

Printed in the United States of America

11 12 13 14 15 16 10 9 8 7 6 5 4 3 2 1

To Shahzad Gill for His Courage and Faithfulness

Contents

Preface

Today is Sunday, May 9, 2010. It is Mother's Day and the thirtieth birthday of my middle son, Johnny—certainly an appropriate combination to celebrate! I just returned from morning Mass and I am so excited I couldn't wait to get to my computer! Why? Because I have been struggling with this book—waiting for God's call and direction—wondering if this book is of Him or just of me. Maybe God is not really calling me to do this. Maybe I just want to do it and I am pushing forward without His blessing. But last night the words started to come to me—at first tentatively and by the end of the evening in a rush. Still, I was not totally pleased with the chapter I had been writing. Then in Mass this morning, Father Foley focused on the work of the Holy Spirit of God and how the Spirit called the early church leaders to closely examine their practices before burdening the Gentiles, new believers who were open to God's spirit, with the same practices. The early church had to listen to the voice and direction of the Holy Spirit. I had been contemplating the future direction of faith community/parish nursing and the priest's words confirmed for me that my thoughts were of the Lord. My mind was flooded with words—with phrases and entire sentences. I pulled out a notepad from my purse and wrote feverishly, afraid that I would not remember all the words and ideas that God was giving me—oh ye of little faith! I was so excited and overwhelmed with His presence as I sat in the pew that I could hardly contain myself.

I was also worried about the preface—what wonderful words could I possibly write that nurses would recognize from the very first page of this book to the last page, that they had read something ordained, blessed, and guided by the Holy Spirit? I heard God call me to tell my story—to share with each of you my familiarity with God's call and the power that call has to transform us, to direct our decisions and actions. You are reading the product of that excitement, that sense of call! It always amazes me, no matter how often it happens, that God chooses me to write—to be a voice to nurses about God's goodness and presence and holiness. Sometimes the call is not as overwhelming as it was this morning. Sometimes I hear it as a gentle voice, a whisper; other times it is a nudge, a sense of rightness. But this morning it was a Hallelujah chorus!

Being obedient to God's direction, I will share with you my call. It is not to be a faith community/parish nurse; rather, it is to be a teacher and writer for nurses about spiritual matters, about God and God's goodness. God has always used my role as a mother to speak to my heart, probably because I can't think of anything more important in this world than to be a good parent, a good mother. When my first son, Adam, was born in 1975 (yes, he will be thirty-five this year and I can't imagine where the years have gone), I had fallen away from the church and from God and was trying to make it on my own without a relationship that I had known since I was a child. Since my childhood, I have been blessed with a vision of Jesus and me as a little girl with long braids, sitting together on a park bench. He has his arm over my shoulder and is looking into my eyes as if I am the only little girl in the world. I am pouring out my heart to Him and He listens like a big brother. Sometimes He gives me advice and direction; sometimes He is just present to me and that is enough. Why I would have ever moved away from this intimate loving relationship, I have no idea. But in His goodness, He called me back and He used Adam's birth to do that.

The Catholic Church offers a baptismal seminar for new parents contemplating baptism for their child. The purpose is to make sure that parents appreciate the significance of their role in nurturing the spirit of their child and teaching by word and deed the love of God. My husband and I met with a very young priest, probably only a few years older than we were at the time. He asked us why we wanted

Adam baptized and we gave him such a poor answer that it shames me to repeat it, but I will. We told the priest that we had been baptized and that our families expected this of us, but in truth we wanted Adam to be free to choose what he wanted to believe in. The foolishness of those words still humbles and embarrasses me. The priest's response was loving and without judgment. He told us that, although our ideas sounded good, we needed to look at the fact that the world would be ready to fill Adam with beliefs, attitudes, and practices that we would not want Adam to adopt, and if he had nothing solid from us by which to compare what the world offered, we might find that what we thought was an enlightened view might leave our precious son with a moral and spiritual vacuum. This young priest sent us away with prayer and a request that we think about what he had said before returning the following week for additional instruction.

That week I could think of nothing else. The Lord used the priest's words and Adam's well-being to speak to me. I was convinced in that week of how far I had moved away from the Lord and knew that it was me who had done the moving. I began to pray again—not a little bit; it seemed as if prayer were constantly on my lips. That summer God introduced me to Charismatic Catholic Christians. I began attending prayer meetings where people prayed in tongues and others interpreted the messages; where participants sang loudly and with joyfulness; where arms were raised in ecstasy! Although I had known the Lord in a personal way as a child, I reaffirmed that relationship and the Lord changed me inside out and is still doing His work in me. I found I was more peaceful and more desirous of prayer and scripture study; I never missed Mass; I felt alive and blissful in a way that I had never experienced before. I can't express how totally transformed I was. I didn't have a horrible story to tell. I wasn't addicted to drugs or alcohol. I had a loving husband and family. I was already blessed. But the transformation inside, within my spirit, was a true metamorphosis. I had always been quiet and shy—I almost never spoke up. No one would ever have described me as bold—but bold I became!

I was so zealous, perhaps even overzealous! I offered to pray with anyone I felt was in need. To give you an example of my fervor, one day

I drove into a service station owned by a Christian fellow who had a marquee on his lot that featured scripture passages. It was a winter's day, brutally cold and snowing. The service attendant, John, came up to my window to ask me what I needed. He looked wretched—he had a terrible cold; his nose was running, he was sneezing constantly, and he was working outside in miserable weather. I remember saying to him, "John, I think you need prayer—let me pray that God heals you today." Without hesitation, John reached in through my car window, we held hands, and I prayed for his healing! Since then I have learned to be more attuned to God's "gentle nudges" in matters like this.

At this time in my life, I was a young faculty member at the University of Maryland School of Nursing and was blessed to work with wonderful women—some were mentors, some were just starting to teach, but all became friends. I shared with them my extraordinary conversion experience and suggested that we should include prayer in our faculty meetings, in our deliberations about students, in everything we did. They were all open to this, and prayer became a regular part of our teaching. This was an anointed time for me—God showered me with grace and blessings. I felt God's presence around me and in me. I heard a distinct call that I needed to write and I obeyed. I started to write, and between 1977 and 1980, I had eight of my works published—all except one focused on the importance of spirituality in nursing. The one exception was a poem titled "A Miracle Come True," which appeared in the *American Journal of Maternal Child Nursing*. The poem was about the miracle of my son, Adam.

There is one other experience I want to share with you to demonstrate my familiarity with God's call. Throughout the 1980s, I felt certain that God wanted me to write a book about spirituality in nursing. I wasn't sure how to break into the book publishing world, but I felt led to contact all the major nursing publishers and offered to be a reviewer of new manuscripts. This gave me the opportunity to impress these editors with my writing skills, to please them with my punctuality in meeting deadlines, and to let them know about my own desire to write. Every publisher included a form to be completed when the review was submitted. This form asked for information about the reviewer and the reviewer's desire to author a book. On every form I always indicated that I wanted to write a book on spirituality in nursing.

In the meantime, moving forward in faith that the book would be published, I was already writing the book. The writing began following a Nurses Christian Fellowship conference that I had attended in New Jersey in 1982. Driving home to Baltimore, I had to pull off the road because I was flooded with the entire outline for *Spiritual Dimensions of Nursing Practice* (a book that was published in 1989) and I had to write it down. I don't mean I received topical headings—I received the entire detailed outline! It just came to me—it was a gift! So, of course, I started writing. I knew it was just a matter of time until God convinced an editor that she could not live without adding a spirituality tome to her roster of books. Finally, in 1988, I received a call from Ilze Raider from Saunders Publishers in Philadelphia. She said that Saunders was willing to take a chance with a book on spirituality, even though they were pretty sure it would be a financial loser. Immediately, I sent her almost the entire book!

So, can you see why I was worried when the words were not coming to me? Can you understand my excitement when I was flooded with words, ideas, phrases, and complete sentences this morning in Mass?

All this is to tell you that I understand God's call—I am living His call on my life. I appreciate and honor His call within the specialty of faith community/parish nursing and I hope His words spoken through me validate the rightness of your call and encourage you to continue responding with your whole heart to whatever God directs you to do, wherever and however He directs you to do it!

Blessings to each of you who read this book!

—Verna

Parish Nursing

Introduction

Now let us turn our attention to you—the reason for this book. Before there were word processors, computers, typewriters, or other implements to write with, there were stories. The collective wisdom of generations has been passed down through storytelling. Stories spark the imagination; they inspire and motivate; they teach and encourage; they correct and challenge. Stories are indeed powerful. And so we have chosen to present the stories of parish nurses—to allow you to hear them describe their journeys in their own voices. Hopefully, you will learn from them, be inspired and motivated by them, and allow your imagination free rein to envision faith community/parish nursing operating in your church and your health care system.

We believe that faith community/parish nursing offers hope to a beleaguered and increasingly inadequate health care system, in which the demands for care—especially long-term care—are outstripping the available resources. There is growing discontent with our medical system. While it is touted as the best in the world technologically, it is criticized for its neglect of the individual. While costs continue to rise, care continues to diminish. Witness the increased interest in and adoption of alternative and complementary medical practices, such as herbal medicine, acupuncture and acupressure, therapeutic touch, crystal therapy, reiki, and reflexology, to name just a few. This trend can be partially explained by the dissatisfaction people feel toward traditional Western, or allopathic, medicine. People want to be cared for in a wholistic manner—to be heard; to share in decision making about their lives; to be loved even when they are unlovable; to be accepted as they are in their brokenness; to be encouraged to delineate their own values, goals, and personal views; and to be recognized as more than a diseased gallbladder or a serious case of depression. Patients want health care providers to see beyond presenting symptoms to the impact of these symptoms on their lives, their work, their capacity to experience joy, their ability to engage in family life, and their experience of spirituality. Patients have always known that they are so much more than the divisible components of body and mind that are the focus of most contemporary medical treatment. Wholistic care recognizes that people are indivisible wholes—fully integrated physical, emotional, intellectual, social, and spiritual beings. Faith community/parish nurses recognize this and respond to it.

An old adage holds that there is nothing new under the sun, just old ideas rediscovered and repackaged. Whether this adage is true or not in general, it is certainly true for faith community/parish nursing with its focus on "caring for" rather than curing. This "new" specialty represents a return to the Judeo-Christian roots of nursing. Jesus focused on the meaning of suffering and the healing of the whole person; He made little distinction between healing of the body, mind, or spirit. His teachings emphasize how the cerebral life of the individual affects health and the power of prayer affects healing. According to G. B. Ferngren, caring for the sick was Christianity's novel contribution to health care.[1] At that time, the pagan community offered no organized care for their sick. The Jewish community provided excellent care for its own, but not for gentiles. The Christian community, on the other hand, offered care not only to Christians but to non-Christians as well. While this was often done in order to convert others to Christianity, it also served a tremendous need and became the forerunner of today's public health system.[2]

Some of the earliest nurses believed that their sole purpose was to honor Christ's commands to minister to the least fortunate among them. They recognized that caring for others extended beyond ministry to physical needs. Their care included providing intellectual and spiritual nourishment, clothing others with human kindness and concern, remembering individuals who had been forgotten or neglected and were no longer cared for and loved, and providing hospitality for people who were homeless or who felt lost in a strange environment. In their ministrations, these nurses saw spiritual meaning in the care they provided. They believed that when they cared for the ill and needy in this fashion, they were serving not only the ill, but God as well.[3]

Over the years, nursing gradually moved away from its spiritual roots. It expanded beyond church-based hospitals and into secular institutions of care. Nursing training, initially controlled by religious orders, came under the purview of state-controlled universities. The twentieth century saw an upheaval in all areas of nursing. Professional organizations were developed to exercise control over nursing practice; educational programs delineated levels of practice and different roles for nurses, depending on their preparation; licensure came about as a way of ensuring nursing competence. Meanwhile, nursing focused increasingly on the scientific and technological advances that were occurring throughout health care and integrated these advances into nursing education and practice. Wholistic care—and especially recognition of the importance of spirituality, faith, and religion to a person's overall health—took a backseat to "high-tech" interventions. For a time, "high touch" had certainly moved out of fashion in the nursing profession.

However, even with these changes, there always remained a cadre of nurses who kept alive the earlier vision and mission of nursing and held fast to the belief that the essence of nursing is to care about and for the whole person. The theme of service and ministry is evident in the writings of many of the twentieth-century nursing leaders as well as many twenty-first-century nursing leaders.

As the twentieth century came to a close, there was growing dissatisfaction among nurses regarding the movement of the profession away from a whole-person focus. Nurses expressed concern that, increasingly, there was little distinction between nursing and medical care. This discontent among nurses led to the development of organizations such as Nurses Christian Fellowship (NCF) and the American Holistic Nurses Association. Both of these organizations focus on the spiritual aspects of health: NCF does so from a Christian perspective and publishes the *Journal of Christian Nursing*; the American Holistic Nurses Association takes this approach from a perspective encompassing other spiritual traditions and publishes the *Journal of Holistic Nursing*.

In the 1980s, Reverend Granger Westberg "rediscovered" church-based nursing and called it *parish nursing*. It is in honor of Reverend Westberg that we use the word *wholistic*, rather than *holistic*. He strongly believed that the *w* was essential to connote "whole person,"[4] which is the focus of the faith community/parish, or congregational, nurse. This ministry began as one strongly connected to and rooted in the Christian faith. However, just as the earliest Christian nursing practice was inclusive rather than exclusive, extending health care to both Christian and non-Christian communities, the concept of faith community/parish nursing has spread beyond the Christian church. In 1998 the American Nurses Association, in collaboration with the Health Ministries Association (HMA), the professional membership organization for nurses in this specialty, developed and published *Scope and Standards of Parish Nursing Practice*. In 2005, this document was transformed into *Faith Community Nursing: Scope and Standards of Practice* in order to embrace a nondenominational, ecumenical perspective.[5] This document points out that the faith community nurse (FCN) bridges two disciplines and thus must be prepared in and responsive to both. "Appropriate and effective practice as an FCN requires the ability to integrate current nursing, behavioral, environmental and spiritual knowledge with the unique spiritual beliefs and practices of the faith community into a program of wholistic nursing care. This is necessary no matter the level of education the nurse has achieved" (p. 4). Let me close this paragraph with a definition of parish nursing that Wendy Walnock, a parish nurse at St. Joseph's Catholic Church in Keyport, New Jersey, uses whenever she is asked to discuss what a parish nurse does and what it means to be a parish nurse. "I define parish nursing very descriptively by saying, 'It reminds me of a peanut butter and jelly sandwich. . . . One slice of bread is the medical aspect (doctors, medical services, etc.), the other slice of bread is the spiritual support (pastors, priests, rabbis, Eucharistic ministers, prayerfulness, etc.), and the parish nurse is the peanut butter and jelly that bring everything together, making it whole!'" Recognizing that the focus of faith community/parish nursing extends beyond Christian theology, we attempted to identify nurses involved in faith community/parish nursing who represent other faith traditions so that we could include their stories as well. Unfortunately, we were less than successful in this outreach effort. We heard of Jewish congregational nurses, but were unsuccessful in obtaining their stories. We sought information from leaders within the parish nurse movement regarding their knowledge and contacts with nurses from non-Christian faith traditions. Reverend Richard Cathell (see Chapter 8) told us about a Buddhist nurse who has completed the required training to be a faith community/parish nurse, but offers her services at an office of elder care lawyers. We received stories from nurses outside the United States. For example, Shahzad Gill, a nurse in Pakistan, shared his story with us, but Shahzad is also Christian. Our attempts to connect with non-Christian nurses in this second edition of Parish Nursing were futile—perhaps, an excellent reason for a sequel!

This book tells the stories of faith community/parish nurses as they make their way through a profession that is still fairly new and still working to achieve acceptance. Many faith communities not only lack a faith community/parish nurse but have not even heard of such a nurse. The road map is certainly better defined than it was in 2002; there are increasing numbers of faith community/parish nurse-coordinators or, as Ruth Syre describes her role, "I am a parish nurse to parish nurses." There are resources and supports available to assist nurses beginning this journey, but for the brand-new faith community/parish nurse, there are still relationships to be developed; connections to be made; assessments to be completed as she/he develops in this role.

The words of the nurses present stories of hearing God's call, of their responses to this call; of their faith that they are doing the "right thing"; of their joys, sorrows, and challenges; and of their quiet determination and dedication as they offer their time and talents to meet the needs of others. Their stories inspired us and we are grateful for the generous spirit of so many nurses. They responded to our questionnaire; they answered countless e-mails; they shared their resources so we might share them with you; they opened their hearts to us, just as they open their hearts to the congregants they serve. We hope that this book honors faith community/parish nurses around the globe and serves as an encouragement to other nurses to respond to that gentle "God nudge" they may be feeling. We hope, too, that the book inspires church members and leaders as well as health care providers and administrators to explore the values and benefits of faith community/parish nursing within their own faith traditions and to the health care system at large.

May God's blessing be upon your ministries!

1. Answering the Call

Meanwhile, little Samuel was helping the Lord by assisting Eli. Messages from the Lord were very rare in those days, but one night after Eli had gone to bed (he was almost blind with age by now), and Samuel was sleeping in the Temple near the Ark, the Lord called out, "Samuel! Samuel!"

"Yes?" Samuel replied. "What is it?" He jumped up and ran to Eli. "Here I am. What do you want?" he asked.

"I didn't call you," Eli said. "Go on back to bed." So he did.

Then the Lord called again, "Samuel!" And again Samuel jumped up and ran to Eli.

"Yes?" he asked. "What do you need?"

"No, I didn't call you, my son," Eli said. "Go on back to bed."

Samuel had never had a message from Jehovah before. So now the Lord called a third time, and once more Samuel jumped up and ran to Eli.

Then Eli realized it was the Lord who had spoken to the child. So he said to Samuel, "Go and lie down again, and if he calls again, say, 'Yes, Lord, I'm listening.' So Samuel went back to bed.

And the Lord came and called as before, "Samuel! Samuel!" And Samuel replied, "Yes, I'm listening."

—I Samuel, 3:1–10[1]

Many of us can identify with young Samuel. We hear a voice calling us—a soft, gentle, but persistent voice. We may not immediately recognize the caller. Maybe we are slow to respond. However, there is something very compelling about this voice and over time we may wonder about the caller's message. Like Samuel, we may sense that we just need to listen. There are, however, other times when the caller is asking us to do more than listen—we are called to change—our behavior, our career, our course in life. Responding is sometimes difficult, sometimes not.

Most nurses who become parish or faith community nurses hear this call and make a choice to listen and respond with a resounding "yes" to God's call in their lives. Many walk away from traditional health care, from higher-paying jobs with greater benefits and more clearly defined boundaries. Other nurses continue to straddle two worlds—the world of nursing within a faith community and the world of nursing within the traditional health care system. All are responding to God as Samuel answered: "I am listening."

This chapter recounts the stories of call experienced by newly contacted parish nurses as well as many of those nurses who participated in the first edition of this book. It is the story of how God's call is being heard by nurses beyond the borders of the United States—in distant places, such as Pakistan, Australia, New Zealand, Europe, and South Africa. For some nurses, the call is to provide service to an individual faith community; to others, the call is to serve other parish nurses; and to still others, the call has been to organize the ministry to serve a broader community. Each nurse hears and responds to God's call in her/his individual way. Let's listen to the stories of parish nurses, hear their voices, and experience their encounters with God.

The first story of call is an incredibly powerful story as it is told by Shazhad Gill, a parish nurse in Pakistan. His call is nothing less than a series of miraculous occurrences as God breaks through to him with the offer and means to first become a nurse and then a parish nurse. Reading this story will prompt a WOW reaction!

It was June or July of 1997—I do not remember exactly. I had passed my matriculation examination and I was thinking about seeking admission to college. I knew that the tuition was beyond my ability to pay and I was sitting alone in a field, thinking about my future. I came to the conclusion that the best I could do to support my family was to work in a factory. While I was thinking about how I would earn money, I saw a man coming toward me, wearing black pants and a blue shirt; he was tall and young, about twenty-eight to thirty years old. He asked me, "Are you a Christian?" "Yes," I replied. He said, "I heard you passed your matriculation examinations with an A+." I told him that was true. He then asked me, "Do you want to become a nurse?" At that time I was very aware of nursing; many of my female relatives were nurses. At that time, in my culture only women became nurses and at that time, nurses were not held in high esteem. Without a second thought, I answered, "Yes, I would like to become a nurse." This man asked me to take him to my home, which I did. I introduced him to my mother and father and while I went to the market to bring something back for our guest, he spoke with my parents. When I returned, they all seemed so happy. A few weeks later a letter arrived from a Christian missionary hospital in Quetta, advising me that I needed to take a written test and be interviewed. The test and interview took place in the Christian Hospital in Taxilla, near Islamabad, Pakistan. My father and I traveled to this place and I took the examination, along with many other candidates, all of whom were from well-to-do families. My sense was that they were all better educated than I was. I thought that I had no chance of being accepted into the nursing program. A month later I was interacting with my friends in our church compound—it was evening when the postman came and gave me a brown envelope with the name of the Christian Hospital in Quetta. I was so excited—I had been accepted into the nursing program! I immediately rushed into the church to pray and say, "Thank you God!" I then went home to tell my family the wonderful news. They were all so happy—all of our neighbors came to share in our joy! On March 20, 1998, I reached the Mission Hospital in Quetta where many missionaries from the UK and the USA came to teach us. I remained there until September 2001. During those 2½ years, I saw very little of my family; I don't know who paid for my education. No one ever asked me for tuition payments and all my needs were met. Without hesitation I have to say that those days were golden days for me and I am so thankful to God. I have also received training in drug abuse prevention. Currently, I work in a government hospital in Islamabad.

I learned about parish nursing and wanted to become such a nurse. Why? I believe nursing is a profession that deals with human beings in times of suffering. The first male nurse was Adam, who cared for his wife, Eve, when she gave birth to the first baby of the world. My Lord and Leader, Jesus Christ, took a bowl of water and a piece of cloth and washed the feet of His disciples—just the way nurses do during morning care for patients. Today nurses need to care for the church, the body of Christ. I believe that when nurses care for the church they are caring for Jesus Christ. I believe that God's plan is for parish nurses to care for individuals, for the church and for nations. The role of the parish nurse is not to minister to a single community but to heal all nations. I call this the advanced role of parish nurses. Just as hospital nurses care for sick people, parish nurses care for sick nations!

In early April of 2009 I was blessed to attend a course on parish nursing that was sponsored by the Nurses Christian Fellowship of Pakistan. Within a week of taking this course I spoke to three pastors about parish nursing and one of those pastors was very interested. I used everything to convince the pastor—prayer, information I had learned at the course, and a commitment to help improve the health of the congregation. He allowed me to speak to the church management. I was given permission to begin my practice but on one condition—that I supply everything that I need. The church could only give me space. I began by taking blood pressures. On June 4, 2009, the pastor invited me to share a cup of tea and he introduced me to thirty church members as the parish nurse. I was given the opportunity to introduce parish nursing to the congregation. The reception was very good—the congregation liked the idea of having a parish nurse.

I feel such delight to be in this role. I have faith in God and I believe He has called me to serve the church community through my profession. Simply put, I am so happy to be a parish nurse and to be responding to God's call.

Carole Kornelis, a parish nurse in Washington State, participated in the first edition of this book. When asked about her experience of God's call, she said:

My call to parish nursing back in 1997 has not changed. In fact, I feel stronger than ever that parish nursing is essential to church/community ministry. I truly believe in a wholistic approach to wellness and have seen the need to assist church members in identifying their need for God's presence as essential when they request healing and peace. I do my work on a personal spiritual basis. I embrace change and am excited to see health ministry continue to grow in our country, knowing that God's love becomes tangible through the caring hands and hearts of parish nurses and community ministers . . . and thus healthier congregations and community members. We need to provide a faith picture of God doing miraculous things! We are called to be obedient to God and to prayer. My prayer is that God meets the deepest needs of healing and wholeness and enables people to experience the abundant life that God promises in scripture.

Michalene King, PhD, RN, the parish nurse coordinator for Wintersville, Ohio, parish families, always knew she wanted to be a nurse. As an adult she also wanted to serve her church community but was unsure how to do this until she heard about parish nursing.

I initially discovered parish nursing at the Urban Mission, an outreach of the Methodist church in Steubenville, Ohio. I went there with my community nursing students and started to volunteer with the parish nurse there. After working for a while, I talked with my pastor, who told me that another nurse was also interested in developing a parish nurse practice in our faith community. I contacted her and we began to develop a plan to start a parish nursing practice. This was the spring of 1997—we did not start the ministry until 1999.

The call of Donna Kremer, MDiv, RN, a Wellstar congregational nurse in Marietta, Georgia, took her from nursing to seminary before focusing on health ministry as a parish nurse.

I have been a nurse (BSN) for over thirty-five years, and have long considered nursing my ministry. In 1994, when my oldest child entered college, I experienced a longing to continue my education. After several months of frustrating inquiries into various graduate specialties—both nursing and non-nursing—a "chance" encounter with a motivational speaker led me to pursue seminary. I say "chance" because I now recognize the fingerprints of God all over this life-changing experience. Two weeks later I was enrolled in seminary.

Over the next six years, I struggled to discern the meaning of my call to seminary and whether or not I wanted to change my self-identification from a nurse to a minister. Although I took numerous Pastoral Care courses and an independent study in Congregational Health Ministry, it was not until I completed an extended unit of Clinical Pastoral Education (CPE) with the urban homeless that I experienced my "epiphany"—the real answer was not "either/or" but "both/and." I then began to articulate my vision for health ministry and earnestly explore opportunities to actualize my calling.

At the same time, I was contemplating transferring my church membership and discussed with the senior pastor how my gifts could best be used in ministry at the new church. To my surprise, he suggested establishing a health ministry. He championed the cause; the leadership and the congregation enthusiastically embraced the ministry.

The reward of establishing relationships through health ministry with members of this congregation continues to be my greatest joy. Health ministry has provided entry into true spiritual intimacy with these wonderful folks.

Elizabeth Pokorney describes an immediate sense of call after reading her church's bulletin.

I was at St. Margaret Mary's Church, in Council Bluffs, Iowa, for Mass, when I opened the bulletin and noticed an insert announcing the start of a parish nursing program in the parish. I had heard about parish nursing about eight years before this and always thought I would like to learn more about it. Well, I feel I was "shoved by the dove" after reading the bulletin insert and called for more information. As we know, all in God's time. Working as a home care and hospice nurse helped me in my endeavor to be a parish nurse.

Sonja Simpson had assisted another parish nurse at a large church where Sonja was a member. She felt drawn to the personal interactions with church members. When Sonja relocated to Arizona with her husband, she became involved in wholistic nursing and spiritual growth. Parish nursing seemed like a natural fit. She asked her minister if she could be the parish nurse and he agreed. This began her wonderful journey that has continued for over ten years. Sonja currently ministers as a parish/faith community nurse in Nebraska, where she serves two different congregations. Sonja believes that, through parish nursing, God affords her the opportunity to practice the true art of nursing.

Yvonne Stock, RN, MS, a parish nurse from Omaha, Nebraska, shares her experience of call—not to a specific faith community but to many communities.

I became interested in exploring parish nursing while doing my daily prayers shortly before leaving for a mission trip to Israel. I was older, but still not "old" in my opinion—approaching seventy—and I asked the Lord where He wanted me to serve. Just before leaving, I visited my home church and talked to the leaders about setting up a parish nurse program and the benefits for the congregation. The pastor said he would send me an e-mail and let me know his decision about having a parish nurse while I was in Israel, but I received none. I returned on a nineteen-hour flight from the mission trip and prayed en route about whether to go to the second day of the parish nurse class the next morning; after all, I had no commitment to serve in my church. After praying, I got up and went regardless of whether I had a parish nurse position or not. I would wait for the Lord for to determine my placement. I graduated in the spring of 2006 from the parish nursing course I had started in 2005. (I missed the first day of class because I was returning from Israel and had to complete that day with the next class.)

My home church still has not asked anyone to become their parish nurse. They have, however, used materials developed by my current employer, CHAMPS (Center for Healthy Aging, Ministries, Programs and Services). Instead of one church, the Lord had something else in mind. I applied for and was hired in the position of parish nurse with CHAMPS.

CHAMPS focuses on healthy aging and sets as its goal to support what older adults identify as important in their spiritual, physical, emotional, social, and financial lives. CHAMPS is designed to be a reproducible model and we work with other churches to assist them in developing their own unique approach to serving the needs of their congregation and community as they age. In the initial partnership phase, CHAMPS has been working with St. Paul's Lutheran, Faith Westwood United Methodist, and St. John Vianney Roman Catholic Church. Our reach is expanding to include at least fifty other congregations located in the Omaha, Nebraska, area.

Ruth Syre, MSN, RN, FCN, wears two hats. She serves as the parish nurse to a small congregation of about fifty members as well as the congregational health coordinator within the Pastoral Care Department of Centra Health System in Lynchburg, Virginia. Ruth describes her coordinator role as being a "parish nurse for parish nurses." She describes her call in this way:

I first heard of parish nursing from a Catholic friend in the late '80s. It left my personal radar for a while, and then resurfaced in 1997. I began reading everything I could about it and corresponding with an educator elsewhere in the state. I told my church family and my own family that this made so much sense to me in a new job with a coworker who just "happened" to be on the planning committee for a new parish nursing course. I was able to be one of the charter students in the Virginia Parish Nurse Education Program in 1998, and have never regretted it for a moment.

Helen Vaughn, FCN, a faith community nurse in New Zealand, shares her experience of call.

Several years ago I read an article in the New Zealand nursing journal, *Kai Tiaki*. I really liked the idea of parish nursing and mentioned it to one or two people. However, personal circumstances prevented me from pursuing it at that time. I did make contact with the New Zealand Faith Community Nurse Association (NZFCNA) and received information from them. About three years ago, I saw that the national conference was to be held in a nearby city, so I decided to attend and find out more. I was convinced that this was the way to go. As I prayed about it, things fell into place. Parish nursing was not a natural role for me, as most of my nursing life has been as a preoperative nurse. So I had to be really sure that this was what God wanted me to do. I have been practicing in the role for a year and I love it!

Jan Marsh, RN, a parish nurse at First Presbyterian Church of Bethlehem, Pennsylvania, emphasizes the role of prayer in discerning a call from God.

I was fortunate to retire early, since my husband had an excellent pension from a large corporation and we both felt that we wanted to serve the church and Our Lord Jesus Christ more fully. Because we had to care for some elderly family members, however, my dream of traveling to distant lands to serve in Christian hospitals for the needy was denied. As I began to pray, I felt God was telling me to "grow where I was planted." I became certified as a parish nurse and then began to implement the role within my church community. My heart is still longing to serve in international areas of severe poverty, but God assures me that I am contributing my gifts to my community.

Sharon Hinton, UMCOR-Health parish nurse consultant and executive director of Rural Nurse Resource, Inc., also emphasizes the importance of prayer in discerning her call to parish nursing.

After praying for guidance for many months, I received a flier in the mail for a parish nurse basic prep course being offered in South Texas. I wanted to attend, but I had two young children and the course was a week long. To my surprise, my husband thought I should attend and offered to take care of the kids in addition to doing his farm work. I needed a recommendation from my church. The pastor thought it was a great idea and an elder who was a retired nurse decided to attend the course with me—not to become a parish nurse, but so that she could better support my ministry. I was amazed! I went to the conference office to ask for support. The assistant to the bishop said that if I felt called to this ministry, the church would pay my expenses. God is amazing. Since that training in 1999, God has continued to open doors and provide for my needs as I serve in this ministry. He paved the way for me to complete the

BSN degree and just when I thought I was finished, a flier for a master's in parish nursing degree arrived! I threw it away and received another one the next day. I gave up and agreed to cooperate with God's larger plan and now have a master's degree in parish nursing and a master's certificate in pastoral studies. The doors continue to open as God guides my ministry to teach others about parish nursing and health ministry.

Eileen Altenhofer, parish care committee chair of Normandy Park Congregational Church in Seattle, Washington, who contributed her story to the first edition of this book, shares how a call can change and yet still keep its original focus of serving God.

I am no longer the parish nurse for my church; however, I still have a keen interest in parish nursing. Life's events mold us in ways that are unexpected and I am finding that perhaps I am no longer meant to be the "goer and doer," but rather to share what I have learned with those who follow in my footsteps.

I am now the parish committee chair. In this role I mentor the current parish nurse and recruit volunteers to help with the program. There has been great evolution in the program at our church.

In the early years of the program, I shared the position of parish nurse with another trained parish nurse, Joan Wieringa. We combined the activities of the lay caregivers of the "Called to Care" Program, which was developed by the Office for Church Life and Leadership of the United Church of Christ, and that of the parish nurse into one program, which we call Parish Care. During this time, the parish nurse was coordinator of the program, which involved working with lay volunteer caregivers. We also performed traditional activities of the parish nurse, which entailed the roles of referral source and liaison with the community resources, health educator, and advocate for healing in the body, mind, and spirit by assisting the pastor in providing spiritual support of the congregational members when making home, hospital, and nursing home visits.

A catalyst for changing the program a bit was that, following my husband's retirement in 1999, I stepped down from the role of parish nurse, but remained a committee member with the responsibilities of preparing bereavement packets, being cofacilitator of our Family Caregiver Support Group, and maintaining our Parish Care Resource Center. At this point, it was decided that we needed to establish the parish nurse as a paid staff position. This would ensure that the program would continue even when we didn't have a nurse in our congregation who was willing and able to be the parish nurse. The Diaconate, which is the board that Parish Care fell under, readily approved this proposal. Their biggest concern was whom they would find to take our place when the time came that both of us were no longer the parish nurses of our church. Joan had decided that she would continue in the role of parish nurse for the time being. That was a great relief and joy for me. I could step down with a clear conscience. Joan took our program to a new level by encouraging all the members of our congregation to feel that they are a part of Parish Care. This concept has been very effective. In times of crisis many members of our congregation willingly step up and offer to help in whatever way they can. This ranges from one gentleman who built a ramp to all who contribute meals, send cards, or who are simply present for one another.

Sharyn Farner, RN, FCN parish nurse, of Messiah Lutheran Church in Halifax, Pennsylvania, describes how others recognized her call before she was aware of it.

Members of the church council approached me about starting a health ministry. Initially I said "no," not wanting the responsibility. Then guilt set in and I began researching parish nursing while I was a nursing student working toward my BSN. A requirement of the nursing program was to develop a community project. I chose to learn more about parish nursing and I shadowed some parish nurses in a distant community. I was absolutely hooked, and knew in my heart that this was for me! Again, the church council approached me and this time I answered with a resounding "yes!" After learning what a parish nurse is able to do, I knew in my heart that this was God's way of tending to His flock by providing health education and support to the congregation. Then, as God would plan it (some would call this a coincidence), I attended a seminar led by Dr. Ruth Stoll who talked about the need for more parish nurses. She announced that a course would begin in the spring. I immediately enrolled in the course and started the Messiah Health Ministry in April 2007.

Mary Jane Fulcher, FCN, in Toledo, Ohio, enrolled in a Congregational Nurse Project seminar, which she found very interesting, but it took a call from the church secretary three years later before she actually answered the call to be a faith community/parish nurse.

Three years ago the Congregational Nurse Project (CNP) Seminar Committee brought Reverend James L. Brooks from Raleigh, North Carolina, to speak on support teams at the annual CNP spring seminar. The content was very well presented and the stories—about how helpful support teams could be to the people working on the team, the congregation, and the person/family being helped—were inspiring. I loved the idea, but it took a call from the church secretary three years later for me to put the knowledge I obtained into practice.

The call for help came to the church from the mother-in-law of the family—she asked if there was anyone who could help her family. The mother and father had five children, all under six years of age. They needed support. The mother was recovering from pneumonia which she contracted just before the birth of their fifth child. Both the mother and baby were rehospitalized after the birth. The extended family members had been helping for over a month and now needed to return to their homes, jobs, and the like. The secretary was overwhelmed with the magnitude of the request and asked me how we should proceed. I immediately remembered the information I had received at the seminar and dusted off the Support Team Handbook. In reviewing the handbook, the concepts from the seminar came alive. I remembered that this should be a team effort. Team members should be asked only to do what they want to do, when they want to do it. The team should work in an organized way and team members should support each other in their efforts. I quickly realized that a support team was exactly what would be helpful to this family.

To start the support team process, on Sunday the pastor from the pulpit asked anyone interested in helping this family to attend a short meeting. Before the meeting, the leader of the support team called the young mother and asked for specific services that the family would find helpful. The mother offered to come to meet the people who wanted to help her family. The mother said she needed help with dinner and with taking care of the children after dinner. The members of the team signed up for what they wanted to do, when they wanted to do it. During the meeting, the important concepts of confidentiality, teamwork, communication, and listening skills were all discussed.

From this experience, I learned the value of being prepared when the time came to step forward to form a team of people who cared deeply and were ready to help a family in need. Team members, as well as the family, gained a real sense of community and caring for one another.

Attending the 2007 CNP Seminar gave me the information, skills, and courage I needed to step forward and say "yes!"

Sometimes the call changes or expands, and God calls the nurse to more. Let's hear the story of Mary Lashley, RN, APRN, a Community Health Board–Certified parish nurse and professor of nursing at Towson University in Baltimore.

I had been a parish nurse for seven years in a small Baptist congregation. It was a typical Sunday evening and I was waiting for the service to begin. There were guest speakers coming that night—men from a mission in downtown Baltimore. They were there to talk about a ministry for the homeless.

I was sitting in the pew with my children, waiting for the service to begin. I thought of the men who had come that evening to speak to us. How disappointing it must be for them to look at the audience and see so few in attendance. There must have been no more than thirty people there that evening and these men had come so far, hoping to recruit support for their organization.

Then it happened: Men began to speak and sing and give powerful testimonies of lives liberated from years of addiction and transformed through the power of Jesus Christ. That is how it all started. It was then I began a journey that changed me and completely challenged my worldview.

Chapter 1

I never considered working with the homeless, much less homeless men, addicts, and ex-convicts. Yet, I was deeply moved by the power of their stories. I was compelled to learn more about this program. It was then that I decided to visit the mission. I could imagine the magnitude of health problems in this population. Since I teach public health nursing at a local university, I saw an immediate opportunity for myself and my students. Still, my view was limited and my intentions self-serving. On top of that, I was scared to death.

As I passed the mission, looking for a place to park, I recalled passing the building years ago and praying "God, please do not let my car break down in this neighborhood." Seeing the men loitering on the street, I remember having thought, "I would never step foot in that place." When I finally made it into the building, I resolved to myself, "I am just taking a few blood pressure readings and getting out of here."

In short, I had found my Nineveh.

That was seven years ago, and how things have changed. Stereotypes have been shattered and my worldview turned on its head. Here are some of the things I have learned:

1. **The story of one of us is the story of us all.** Getting to know these men has made me realize that we have so much in common and are more similar than we are different.

2. **Do not let the fact that you have no idea what you are doing stop you!** I confess that about 80 percent of the time, I have no idea what I am doing! I have been stretched so far—I have served on the Board of Directors, written grants, directed an oral health program that has impacted over a thousand individuals and has received nearly a half million dollars in funding, led a committee to develop an addictions recovery program for women, and been interviewed on TV and radio. And all I ever intended to do was take a few blood pressure readings!

   But God had another plan and I am so glad He did. He equips us for the work He has called us to do. And He sends others to stand alongside us and take up our burdens when we are weary. As we submit to His will and place our trust in Him, suddenly the impossible begins to look possible. And our faith journey is propelled to a whole new level.

3. **If you are faithful to what God has called you to do, good things will come to you.** We do not have to manipulate events or circumstances to get what we want. With some projects, we had reached the end of the road. Our funding sources were exhausted and we saw no options. Yet, God opened new opportunities just when we were ready to pack it in and head home, and brought the right people at the right time to meet our need. When your work is centered on Him, you will give what little you can give and do the little you can do. But then the most amazing thing will happen. God will step in and He will do what you cannot do. He will do what you cannot even imagine. And where does that leave you? You stand back and watch your faith soar!

4. **God will infuse into you His deep and profound love for the people He has called you to serve.** Out of this love, you will be compelled to respond and make a difference. Before you know it, you will find yourself immersed in your calling, living out His love for others in your passions and pursuits.

5. **Finally, you will venture into the unknown, thinking you are bringing hope and healing to others.** But in the process you will soon find that you are the one who is being healed—healed in the broken places in your heart.

Truly, it is great to be on the winning team. It just doesn't get better than this!

Carole Edlan, DMin, RN, director of the RCIA process at the Cathedral of St. Joseph the Workman in La Crosse, Wisconsin, and a chaplain for the county jail ministry, shares her story of call, which arose out of her own experiences with pain and recovery from a near-fatal accident.

On a gray Saturday afternoon, December 19, 1992, I was standing in the doorway of a convenience store waiting while my husband finished filling the gas tank of our automobile. I had planned to ask him if he wanted anything to eat or drink on the last leg of our trip home. We had just completed a three-hundred-mile journey, visiting both of our mothers at opposite ends of the state of Wisconsin, bringing them their Christmas gifts and bags of assorted food. We had gathered with the immediate family of children and grandchildren a few weeks earlier, so I was pleased that now I had six full days to reflect on the ministerial aspects of the approaching Christmas season and the duties I had at my parish church. The 19th of December was also our firstborn's birthday, which made it a special day.

As I stood in the doorway of the store, suddenly the driver of an automobile, which had been parked in the front of the store, shifted the car into reverse and backed up at what appeared to some observers to be at an accelerated pace. This information was given to me after the fact, as I did not see him or hear anything until he collided with an automobile parked at the gas pump nearest to the store, smashing its front fender and grill. Without slowing down, he continued driving backwards in an altered course directly toward me. The idea that he would continue to operate the vehicle and keep on coming toward me seemed impossible. Never once did I think that he would keep his foot on the gas or that he would actually hit me. There was no time to decide what to do. I had no place to run. My entire body was frozen in a state of fear and disbelief. The car continued, jumping over the front step of the store and crashing into me. I was stunned, shocked, and terrified. The unbelievable had become a horrible reality.

In the twinkling of an eye, the car smashed into me, flinging me into the store, where I found myself lying on the floor, surrounded by broken glass, crushed cans of soda and beer, the contents of the shattered containers flooding the area. The car ended up on top of me with the engine still running, allowing gas and noxious fumes to spew over me. "Lord, what has happened? One minute I was standing and now I am flat on my back on the store floor. My legs. I can't feel my legs. Stay with me, Lord. I don't want to die yet. I have so much to do. I need your help."

The customers in the store looked at me lying on the floor under the car with helpless expressions on their faces. My head and part of my shoulders were visible. How could they help? One old woman took my hand and held it firmly while I called out to the Lord for help. I looked up and saw my husband's terrified face as he ran into the store and saw me under the car. "Is she dead?" he shouted with great fear in his voice. He could not get near me. Firemen, policemen, and the ambulance crew arrived and somehow removed the car from on top of me and got it out of the store. I told myself I needed to stay awake. Somewhere I had read that if you stayed alert when you're involved in an accident, you would have a better chance of survival. I did not want to take any chances, so I was determined to stay awake. As I tried to wait patiently for some kind of help, my whole body seemed to want to contract into a fetal position. However, that was impossible as my legs were completely mangled and crushed. "My God, my God, why have you forsaken me?" (Matthew 27:46b). Finally, the paramedics secured my legs with splints for the ambulance ride to the nearest hospital. It all seemed so impossible. One minute I was filled with contentment and wholeness, the next minute agony and brokenness had taken its place. Prayer was first and foremost in my mind and on my lips. "I want to be your servant, Lord. Let me live."

I did indeed live and, in reflecting over the past months and years of recovery, I have come to a new understanding of the gift of life and the vital aspects granted by that gift. To get to that point, I had to do a great deal of coping with crisis and learning about myself. For many years, I was under the great misconception that I was in total control of my life and my destiny. The fallacy of that thinking came to me very quickly as I awakened from the first of my eight surgeries. Without a moment's hesitation, I surrendered myself to the loving embrace of Jesus. I freely gave him control over every aspect of my life. The smug pride that I had always had in thinking I was in charge of events in my life vanished quickly. The very act of relinquishing control to the Lord was extremely freeing and helped remove the fear I had about dying. Clinically, that was still a real possibility, but I had lost the fear of that mortal reality. I felt a peace come over me that enabled me to concentrate on healing, rather than on negative thoughts of death. A warm glow seemed to encapsulate my body with a protective layer of love. I felt doubly blessed with a peace of mind and spirit along with the warmth of the love of the Lord in my heart.

Carole learned many lessons during those years of recovery: Her relationship with God intensified, her prayer life took on new importance, and she developed a new attitude and gratitude for life and living. The lessons painfully learned throughout this period of suffering and healing infuse her ministry of faith community nursing. When confronted with congregants who are asking "Why?" and struggling to find a reason to go on, Carole can fully empathize—she was there!

In recounting the stories of call, we have come full circle. We began with the amazing story of Shazhad Gill and we now share the equally amazing story of Becky Seymour, RN, congregational health ministries coordinator and educator at Memorial Hermann Baptist Beaumont Hospital in Beaumont, Texas. Like Shazhad, Becky describes two separate stories of call. The first call, a call to nursing, occurred with the death of her baby daughter, Sarah Beth. Seventeen years after becoming a nurse, feeling content and satisfied in her nursing position in a Labor and Delivery Department, Becky "heard" about parish nursing and was on the lookout for a nurse to fill a parish nurse position. She did not give a thought to seeking that position herself—why would she? She had just received a day position in Labor and Delivery. Read on and see how the chance finding of a sermon written by her grandfather in 1957, the year of Becky's birth, confirmed God's call to Becky to become a parish nurse! Listen to Becky's words:

I was called into the profession of nursing after the death of my daughter, Sarah Beth. Sarah Beth was born too early and weighed only two pounds and fourteen ounces. She struggled through her short life, but as she did, many lives were changed through the experience. As I watched the nurses and doctors work with little Sarah Beth, I saw something I had never witnessed before. I saw the core of true nursing. The nurses were so kind and gentle with Sarah Beth and always included my husband and me while they cared for her. Sarah Beth lived for only six weeks before she went to be with the Lord. I felt a calling to nursing—to give to others what I had experienced. I worked in Labor and Delivery for over seventeen years. One night as I was walking across the great room in our church, a professor from the local university called me over. She began to tell me about a friend of hers who was looking for a parish nurse-coordinator. I had never heard of parish nursing before and asked her to explain it to me. She began by telling me how nurses were using their professional skills in a ministry for the Lord within their own faith communities. I remember thinking that the ministry of parish nursing seemed to be a great way to reach and educate faith communities, and I asked her: With such a need in our churches for education, why hasn't this been done before? I explained that I had finally received a day position in Labor and Delivery and wasn't looking for a new job, but if I found someone who might be interested in parish nursing, I would pass the information along. I went home that night and didn't sleep a wink. I just couldn't get my mind off parish nursing and why I hadn't thought of it before. What an awesome way to show the love of God!

The next morning I called my educator friend who had told me about the parish nursing job, and I told her that I would like to learn more. Laughing, she said, "I thought you would. You have a 2:30 meeting scheduled with Chaplain Cross today." She told that she felt God urge her to call me over to tell me about the position—and that when God tells you to do something you'd better do it!

I met with Chaplain Cross that afternoon and I told him I would pray about the job and if I found someone who was interested in it I would let him know. I just didn't want to walk away from the facility where I had worked for so many years to start a program that I didn't know anything about.

That evening, as I was cleaning my house, I was sitting on the floor in front of my TV stand. When I pulled out some papers, a small packet of paper fell into my lap. I knew instantly that it was one of my grandfather's sermons. My grandfather had been a preacher for about forty years and he always typed his sermons on small pieces of paper, and made little packets that would easily fit into his Bible. As he preached, he could always go back to his main scripture because of the placement of this small informational packet with his sermon outline on it.

As I picked up the sermon, I turned it over and on the back was written, "High School, 1957." Amazingly, that was the year I was born; he must have been the keynote speaker for a high school graduation that year using this particular sermon. One other touching part of finding this sermon is that there were no other sermons with it, and I really don't know how it got there. I have all of his sermons carefully stored away to give to my nephew, who is now a preacher. I just couldn't believe that the title of the sermon, "The Parting of the Ways," seemed to be directed right toward me. I felt a presence around me as I opened the sermon packet and I was so overwhelmed, just as if God Himself were sitting right next to me. Ezekiel 2:23 was the scripture my grandfather used for this particular sermon: "The King of Babylon stood at the parting of the ways at the road, at the fork of two roads, to use divination: he shakes the arrows, he consults the images, he looks at the river." My grandfather wrote, "When you have been walking or driving in the country, you sometimes come to two roads branched away from the one you are on, like the two arms of the letter Y. As you stand questioning which one to take—for the one would take you where you wanted to go and the other would take you away from it—that spot where you stood uncertain was the parting of the ways." I was already in tears and feeling such a tug to call Chaplain Cross, but I sat there and read the rest of the sermon. The sermon was full of examples about how different people stood in the uncertain place and were asked to make a decision that would virtually change their lives. One example, in particular, really spoke to me. My grandfather wrote, "I read of a dog who had lost his master and ran seeking him here and there until he came to where the way parted; then he was seen to stand perplexed for a while, but at last, without hesitation, he took the right road and trotted off. Why? He had found the way his master had gone, and he knew that if he also went that way he would be sure to come upon his master . . . as he did. So will you young people, if you take the way of the Lord Jesus Christ, you will be certain to take the right way. It is a way of prayer, love, trust, truth, and joy."

After reading this part of the sermon I knew that God was calling me to a new service in Him. I knew that my grandfather was right that the way I should take was one of prayer, love, trust, truth, and joy. I prayed a prayer that I will never forget, "Lord I will follow you wherever You lead me. Give me the peace that I need to know this is what You want me to do and thank you for calling me to another new ministry for you. What a privilege this is."

The next morning I called Chaplain Cross and asked him if I could speak with him. I told Chaplain Cross that I was experiencing a great impression of change about to happen to me concerning my current job. He told me that God might be speaking with me, preparing me for this new position. Chaplain Cross saw something in me and in my testimony, and he told me that he would like to offer the coordinator's position to me. I told him that I would take the position, that I considered this a ministry and not a job, and he totally agreed with me.

Chaplain Cross gave me a brief history about the preparations for the new parish nursing program. For two years prior to ever meeting me, the hospital was budgeting for my position. Several nurses interviewed for the position, but he was unable to find the right person, someone he felt was "called" to fill this position. He told me he felt I was the one God was calling to head up the new parish nurse program. Right after our meeting, Chaplain Cross took me to my new office. As I walked into this office, I saw an empty desk, a pen, a writing tablet, and a computer. In the corner, I saw an empty filing cabinet. Chaplain Cross told me that I was to develop the parish nurse program to cover all of Southeast Texas. I felt a little overwhelmed, but quickly remembered that God had called me to this ministry and it was His ministry, not mine. Now we have over 160 faith communities working in our faith community program with fifty-four trained faith community nurses. God has supplied our needs and we are growing every day. The way has not always been easy, but knowing I am in the exact place God wants me is so fulfilling.

The scripture is the place I found my answer and I know that is where anyone else can find the answers to all of their questions. Although God packaged His word in a very heart-tugging package for me, he might not do that for everyone. I just know that the probability of that sermon written the year I was born, speaking about the parting of the ways, and written for an educational event falling in my lap at that time . . . well, I will just say I know it was the Lord's doing.

We end with one last story, from Shirley Branch, a parish nurse in Houston, on the occasion of her receipt of the Woman of the Year award from Fifth Ward Missionary Baptist Church.

My steps have been ordered. You can see a drag in my step, but yet I march on. My life was in a valley and I felt I had no worth. How would I give back? The word faith kept coming up in my mind over and over. I found a new way to restore my joy by touching the lives of others once again.

I remember saying to my church congregation on my parish nurse dedication, "I didn't know there was an educational program for a church nurse." But a faith community nurse is much more than being a church nurse. It is touching people—mind, body, and spirit—the whole person.

Faith nursing guides my path and with years of wisdom I am able to soar like an eagle. I have seen much from my rock. I now see with a new vision. I have always cared about helping people and I now have a different way of doing just that.

Faith nursing comes from your heart and very seldom is there any pay. It is listening and helping people to improve their lives. It is bringing education to your neighborhood in a way that your neighbors will listen and understand. It is looking at their needs and finding resources that they can use. It is organizing events to bring services and attention to their needs.

The faith community is our extended family and extends us all. For my mother, faith nursing is having Jannie Moore's Comfort Ministry. Her diaper ministry is dedicated especially to the seniors and disabled. It is going green to save green. It keeps them dry, while keeping their expenses low so that they have money at the end of the month for food and medicine. Our health team also recycles gently used clothes, walkers, and wheelchairs. Faith nursing is just being there and daring to care.

There are many other stories from many other parish nurses—but the stories recounted in this chapter clearly show that nurses who choose to work with faith communities do not do so for the money, prestige, or power, but to serve God and God's people. They are responding to a call from God to love, to serve, and to make themselves available to His flock.

Indeed, God is awesome. Gently and persistently He is calling His nurses. Some He speaks to directly; some He speaks to through dreams; some He speaks to through pain and discouragement; and others He speaks to through other nurses. Each hears His call and responds—not always knowing what this new uncharted journey will hold, but moving forward in faith nonetheless. Before going on to Chapter 2, where we explore what God is calling nurses to, it is fitting to end this chapter with the words of a hymn titled "The Summons," a summation of God's call to nurses and their response.[2]

Will you come and follow me if I but call your name?
Will you go where you don't know and never be the same?
Will you let my love be shown? Will you let my name be known,
Will you let my life be grown in you and you in me?

Will you leave yourself behind if I but call your name?
Will you care for cruel and kind and never be the same?
Will you risk the hostile stare should your life attract or scare?
Will you let me answer prayer in you and you in me?

Will you let the blinded see if I but call your name?
Will you set the prisoners free and never be the same?
Will you kiss the leper clean and do such as this unseen,
and admit to what I mean in you and you in me?

Will you love the "you" you hide if I but call your name?
Will you quell the fear inside and never be the same?
Will you use the faith you've found to reshape the world around,
Through my sight and touch and sound in you and you in me?

Lord your summons echoes true when you but call my name.
Let me turn and follow you and never be the same.
In Your Company I'll go where Your love and footsteps show.
Thus I'll move and live and grow in you and you in me.

2. Called to Serve

Ministry of Presence, Word, and Action

Parish nursing is a unique practice model in that nurses are called on less for their "hands-on" skills and much more for their "being with" skills. The literature that describes parish nursing usually focuses on specific functions fulfilled by the nurse. There are a variety of descriptors with great overlap among writers. For instance, Granger Westberg used the term "minister of health" to describe the parish nurse and suggests four major functions: (1) health educator; (2) personal health counselor; (3) trainer of volunteers; and (4) organizer of support groups. Since Westberg's original work, three functions have been added: (1) referral agent and liaison with congregational and community resources; (2) integrator of faith and health; and (3) health advocate.[1] We believe that all seven of these functions are part of three overlapping ministries:

- a ministry of presence, referring to the nurse's ability to "be with" a person and/or a family in need and to demonstrate—without words—love, compassion, and understanding;

- a ministry of action, referring to "how the nurse does what is done" and speaks to the very essence of who the nurse is; and

- a ministry of word, referring to all that the nurse says to the congregation in the way of education, advice, and advocacy.[2]

When nurses focus on all three ministries at once, they are a powerful combination and go to the heart of genuine caring. Toward the end of the first chapter we heard the remarkable story of Becky

Seymour's call to parish nursing. We begin this chapter with another of Becky's stories—this time of how she herself was ministered to by a parish nurse, Pat Olin, who demonstrated the three ministries of presence, word, and action.

My story of becoming a parish nurse is not like anyone else's story. My director thought that since I was going to be reaching so many nurses in Southeast Texas that I should take the basic preparation course from someone special. He sent me from Beaumont, Texas, all the way to Milwaukee, Wisconsin, to take the course from Ann Solari-Twadell and Mary Ann McDermott. I was so excited about taking the course, but to add Marquette University to the plan made it even more exciting.

I arrived late that day and settled into the dorm, only to meet some of my new classmates and we went to dinner. After that I attended the opening night of our program and met the rest of the twenty parish nurse students. I then returned to my dorm room and fell asleep with aspirations of being the best parish nurse ever.

I awoke the next morning with an excruciating pain in my right eye. It felt as if someone were sticking a sharp knife through the center of my eye. I was not oriented to the room and I could not find my cell phone. I entered the hallway and thought that if I could get to the elevator, someone would see me and help me. The elevator doors opened and I heard a sweet voice say, "What is wrong?" I told her that I didn't know but that I was in severe pain and I needed help. She told me she was Ann Solari-Twadell and that she was going to call someone to help me. She helped me sit down on the floor because I couldn't see anything, due to the severe pain. If I opened my left eye, it hurt worse so I just kept both of them closed.

The coordinator of the program was Pat Olin. She helped me get to an acute care center and they immediately told her to take me to the hospital. Once I was seen by the physician, I was told that I needed to give someone my power of attorney and that I should notify my family because he thought I had a brain aneurysm. I was still in severe pain and he told me he couldn't give me anything because he wanted to do an emergency CT scan of my brain. I was so scared and here I was with the lady I really hadn't met, except for the fact that she was driving me around to get me help. I tried to reach my husband, but he was driving senior adults of my church to a camp and he didn't have his cell phone. I asked Pat to call my pastor, and once she reached him she gave me the phone. That is when I truly lost it. I started crying and just hearing his voice I realized how far away from home I was with no one I knew and that at any moment I could be sitting at the feet of Jesus. I told him that I was told to give my power of attorney to Pat and that he needed to locate my husband as soon as he could. He prayed with me and told me he would do whatever I needed done. The doctor told me that if they found something in the CT scan then they would most likely do surgery immediately and I needed to get things in order. All of this was happening so fast around me—I couldn't see anyone and I was in such pain that it was hard to focus on the severity of what was happening. Pat was so wonderful with me. She was my first experience of a parish nurse. She prayed with me, held my hand when I broke down, and held me close to her. I learned so much about parish nursing from her acts of kindness and love. I will never forget all that she did for me. That was Pat's first class to coordinate and I had taken her totally away from her first experience.

As I laid on the CT scan bed, I started to question why I was there and why God had called me away from my secure job as a labor and delivery nurse to travel all the way to Milwaukee to be incapacitated on this bed. I felt a response back from God, telling me, "All is well and I will take care of you. You don't need anyone else because I am with you." I just kept feeling that impression from God: "I am with you."

Later that afternoon I was told that the CT scan was negative for an aneurysm, but they still didn't know what was causing the swelling and pain. They did more tests and finally gave me some pain medication, but through all the testing I missed the second day of class, as did Pat.

As I look back at all that happened to me that day, I realized that several lessons were learned. First of all, God is in control. No matter what I think should happen, He is in control of my life, His ministry, my education, and my health. The second thing that I learned was what parish nursing was all about—that is to use our professional skills in a ministry for the Lord. Because of Pat's training as a nurse, she was able to keep me informed with all that was happening along with helping me make the right decisions related to my care. She was my advocate when I couldn't speak, a source of comfort when I had my meltdown, my guide as we walked together when I could not see. She was the extension of God's hand to me in a very faraway place at a very scary time in my life.

The next day I was a bit better, and I actually attended class. When I walked in, Ann Solari-Twadell was teaching. She stopped, told everyone who I was, and they turned and stood and clapped for me. I didn't know that the entire time I was gone the first day, my sweet parish nursemates were lifting me up in prayer and planning a way to care for me once I returned to them. I really didn't need much care after that second day and I finished the course with one eye. I lost partial vision in my right eye for about a year. My diagnosis was optic neuritis. The physicians told me that they were not going to release me to fly back home until the next week, but God also worked that out for me. I returned to the doctor after four days and he told me that the swelling was going down and that he thought it was safe for me to return home.

On the way home, I had time to think about all the things that happened to me. I felt that something mighty and awesome was about to happen with the new parish nurse ministry that God was starting in Southeast Texas. Instead of being nervous about building the program, I knew I just needed to turn it over to God and let Him build the ministry His way. He has never let me down and I know, even when I can't see, that He is there for me. To God be the glory for the great things He has done!

Wow—what else can be said about Becky's introduction to parish nursing through the ministering of Pat Olin!

Let's hear how other parish nurses describe their service in terms of the seven functions: health educator; personal health counselor; trainer of volunteers; organizer of support groups; referral agent and liaison with congregational and community resources; integrator of faith and health; and health advocate. Box 2.1 illustrates the functions of the parish nurse as the nurse provides the vital link between the

Functions of the Parish Nurse

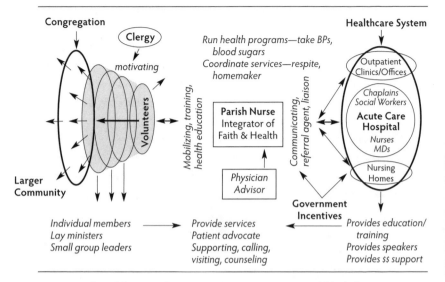

Box 2.1 Adapted from Koenig, H. G., & Lawson, D. M. (2004). *Faith in the future: Healthcare, aging, and the role of religion.* Philadelphia: Templeton Foundation Press.

secular (health care system) and the sacred (congregation). As we discuss each of these functions, we encourage you to refer to this figure.

Health Educator

Every article and book written about parish nursing highlights the function of health educator. Knowledge empowers people. Equipped with adequate understanding, individuals are able to make good health-related decisions. These decisions include ways to preserve health through diet, exercise, and stress management; ways to manage health problems to minimize pain, discomfort, and disability; and ways to live with chronic health problems so that life continues to be a journey of joy and meaning.

In a 2003 article by Medvene et al.,[3] the researchers report on a study involving seventeen faith communities. Two hundred forty-eight (69 percent) of the congregants who started the program completed it. Of the program completers, 83 (33 percent) had an advance directive prior to the program and 140 (56 percent) had a directive after completion. One hundred eighty-six of the completers discussed directives with family members. Overall, 89 (36 percent) of the 248 program completers revised an existing directive or signed one for the first time. Age was positively related to having signed/revised a directive before taking the program. Fear that advance directives would be used to deny medical care was negatively related to signing both prior to the program and after program completion, and contributed to participants' reluctance to sign directives.

All the nurses who shared their stories with us mentioned the importance of conducting blood pressure screenings. A rudimentary nursing procedure serves as an entrée not only into the lives of parishioners but also into the church community itself.[4] Most nurses establish a bimonthly or monthly blood pressure screening regimen, usually following one of the Sunday worship services. Many parishioners who would never voluntarily bare their souls to another find that through the blood pressure screening they are free to share what is most troubling to them. While the nurse is collecting valuable health information, much teaching is conducted at the same time.

Sonja Simpson, RN, MSN, AHN-BC, a parish nurse in Grand Island, Nebraska, who serves two congregations—Messiah Lutheran ELCA and First Presbyterian Church, discusses the importance of the three blood pressure clinics that she holds every month—one at each of the two congregations she serves and one at a senior apartment complex, which is done as an outreach program for one of the congregations she serves.

The blood pressure clinics are a gold mine for connection to a person. The simple act of taking a blood pressure and listening to the words the person might say about her/his blood pressure reading provides a great opportunity to assess other issues of concern. Once people get the sense that they have an opportunity for connection and information, it becomes something much greater than just a blood pressure clinic. I call it my time of "hearing stories."

Education is such an important function of the parish nurse that it is difficult to isolate specific "teachable moments." Most nurses who shared their stories with us identified the many ways that they educate. For instance, there is the informal, one-on-one contact, in which the nurse has the opportunity to teach while performing another task, like screenings for blood pressure, diabetes, pulmonary function, and cholesterol levels; flu-shot administration; or participation in health fairs. Health education is also provided through educational seminars that are initiated by the parish nurse for the congregation. The parish nurse chooses the topics of these seminars after conducting and analyzing a needs assessment for the congregation.[5] Sometimes the nurse is the teacher; other times the nurse invites an expert from the community to share information with parishioners. Topics run the gamut from health care proxies and funeral planning to aging well issues, date rape/abstinence, bereavement, biblically based weight control programs, CPR classes, wholistic heart health, male/female communication, stress, and hope. This is just a sampling of the types of presentations that are being given in churches where parish nursing is operational.[6] Buijs and Olson[7] believe that the parish nurse has an important role to play in providing education for families with young children.

In addition to the informal teaching and the formal seminars, parish nurses also fulfill the health educator function through the development and distribution of written materials, through church bulletin inserts, and through the maintenance of resource centers stocked with both nurse-developed materials and those provided by professional organizations, such as the American Heart Association. Eileen Altenhofer determined that the need was great for bereavement support and education. She developed bereavement follow-up packets for any congregational member(s) who had recently experienced a loss. These packets contain information regarding what grief feels like; how to cope with loss; how to answer the questions of a child about death; how to help a child deal with death; a list of community resources, including support groups; and literature on the grieving process. This packet of information is followed by actions, such as sending sympathy cards to the family, making telephone calls at intervals of one month, six months, and one year; offering special support programs during the holidays; and presenting bereavement and loss services at the church.

Sharon Hinton extends the role of educator beyond the boundaries of her congregation. Let's listen to her story:

I planned to serve my small rural congregation in Texas, but God had bigger plans. I serve multiple congregations and now teach parish nurses and parish nurse-educators. I provide informational support and encouragement to parish nurses nationally. I still have my original motto of being "accessible, approachable, and available," but I have expanded that motto to include "encouraging, educating, and nurturing wholistic health ministry." My ministry includes a local United Methodist congregation and a Hispanic Assembly of God congregation, where I have promatoras (an outreach worker in a Hispanic community who is responsible for raising awareness of health and educational issues). I just love my promatoras! I am so impressed with their excitement for serving their congregations and communities. I find great joy in developing and teaching the program to them. As a result of the skills they have learned and are implementing, they have already intervened with two congregants who had dangerously high blood pressures and have assisted in the care of many other church members.

Personal Health Counselor

Although the parish nurse function of personal health counselor overlaps significantly with the teaching role, counseling is almost always provided in a personal encounter between a faith community member and a parish nurse, or a family and a parish nurse. Counseling certainly entails offering information, but the individual or family's need usually requires much more than a mere factual exchange and calls for dealing with lifestyle issues, as well as emotional and spiritual concerns that complicate health care issues.

In the following vignette we hear a story recounted by Kay Hurd, a parish nurse in New Jersey. Kay's story is important on many levels—certainly in describing the parish nurse's counseling role, but also in illuminating the importance of that role in responding to a major health issue that has physical, emotional, and spiritual implications.

I have worked over twenty years with victims of domestic violence and took the Clinical Pastoral Unit education to be able to address the spiritual needs of the victims. Forgiveness becomes a major problem when it comes to domestic violence. One in five families in churches is experiencing emotional and/or physical abuse, so when I work with the victims of abuse, I frequently focus on spiritual issues. My experience is that after the trauma, spiritual issues are the most important ones to address. These women have lost faith in God, their image that they are children of God, and thus valued human beings. They feel shame and guilt. They have often lost hope and develop depression in grief and mourning.

A girl I was working with was nineteen years old. She had three children less than three years of age and was pregnant with her fourth child. She had been abused since childhood and could only be described as having the flattest affect I have ever seen. Her soul was so lost that her eyes were "dead." My role was to work a few times with her while I found a placement with a family who would take her in, along with her children, on a long-term basis, and would see that she received the long-term psychiatric care she needed. Although I had additional training, I certainly believe that identifying victims of domestic violence and referring them to the appropriate professionals is well within the role of the parish nurse. This is an issue that is swept under the rug in many churches because, too often, the abuser is a board member and the largest contributor to the church. However, domestic violence is not a function of social status or education—PhDs batter at the same rate as high school dropouts. Pastors as well as parish nurses need training in this area because the spiritual issues are so big and difficult to handle and a referral system needs to be in place for team intervention. This is a problem—many times hidden or overlooked—that must be addressed. It doesn't go away.

Trainer of Volunteers

We believe that of all the functions of the parish nurse, the training of volunteers may prove to be the most important service to the health care system as we move forward in this century. Currently, the health care system is struggling to provide adequate care and to contain costs. In 1966, when the Medicare program was first put in place, the total cost of the program per year was less than $5 billion. By 1980 it had increased to $38 billion, and by 1998 it had increased to over $200 billion per year. In 2010 the Medicare budget was projected to be $510 billion per year.[8] As the number of older adults in the population starts dramatically increasing after 2011, when 70 million baby boomers begin moving into the over-sixty-five age range, projected growth and Medicare expenditures may swamp the health care system's ability to provide for all of them. Bear in mind that this is prior to the rapid growth in the elderly population projected to occur after 2011. Many would conclude that our medical system is broken. How, then, will this system now teetering on the brink of collapse respond as the numbers of elderly increase from 35 million currently to over 70 million in a few decades, along with a growing number of health problems, most of which are chronic conditions requiring a great deal of care?

There is a movement toward volunteerism or lay mobilization that is occurring across the country in many churches. This movement is about the Spirit of God working through His people to strengthen the Lord's work.[9] Parish nurses are in a wonderful position to mobilize and train church members of all ages. These volunteers are motivated by the highest goal to serve and honor their God by assisting one another and are the key resource within the church. They need to be utilized more fully. Furthermore, volunteering helps people to stay both mentally and physically healthy, according to a growing body of research in this area.[10]

Marianne Parker describes mobilizing volunteers as a three-step process: invite, ignite, and unite. This process goes beyond the creation and maintenance of a telephone-calling list of potential volunteers. The *invite* step involves giving potential volunteers a clear vision of how they can help and their unique role in the health care ministry process. The parish nurse must recognize that volunteer-ministry experiences serve to highlight and uplift the personal journeys of each volunteer.[11] The parish nurse must honestly value each volunteer and believe that each one is part of God's gift to the faith community.

At the heart of lay ministry are two key relationships—between the volunteer and God and between the volunteer and the parish nurse. Relationships require personal investment and regular tending. Although the invitation to lay ministry can be made through many avenues, including newsletters, church bulletins, pulpit invitations, and small group presentations, there is nothing that takes the place of a personal invitation with its power to communicate relationship and connection. An article in the *Catholic Review* quotes a study conducted by the Georgetown University Center for Applied Research in the Apostolate (CARA). This study profiled Catholics in the Washington, D.C. Archdiocese and confirmed that "being invited" is by far the major reason why Catholics become active in their parish. Furthermore, the study contends that if invitations to lay ministry from fellow parishioners and pastors were extended more, it would translate into at least a 10 percent increase in volunteers willing and even eager to contribute their skills and experience.[12]

As the parish nurse participates in recruiting volunteers, it is essential for the nurse to listen for the message beyond the spoken words. Sometimes a response of "no" may require negotiation and clarification about exactly what is expected of someone who volunteers. The minister must fully support the nurse's efforts to mobilize volunteers and, in particular, preach regularly from the pulpit on the importance of volunteering as the role and responsibility of every Christian. According to Jesus, "Love thy neighbor" was a close second to the first commandment of "loving God." The Apostle John equated these commands: "How can you love God, if you cannot love your fellow man right in front of you?"

Step 2 of the mobilization process is *ignite*, which focuses on training to build essential skills so that volunteers can succeed in their ministry settings. Training is needed so that those who volunteer their time learn the following skills:

- how to listen to others

- how to support others

- how to help the sick and disabled

- how to encourage independence among people with chronic illnesses and disabilities

- how to help the sick and disabled help others

All these skills are considered part of nursing, but in the face of a nursing shortage, volunteers, under the guidance and supervision of the faith community/parish nurse, can provide many of these skills to their fellow parishioners. These services will help to maintain the chronically ill elderly in their homes, give them a sense of vision and purpose for their lives, and decrease the strain on the increasingly limited resources of the health care system.

Using the acronym TRAIN, Parker describes the igniting phase in the following manner:

- Teach the content in a manner and within a time frame that values the experiences and other commitments of the volunteers.

- Respect the time, talents, gifts, passions, questions, learning style, and ideas of the volunteers.

- Actively involve people during training. The nurse must model the ability to step out of a person's comfort zone and consider new behaviors and ways of interacting.

- Ignite a renewed sense of God's call to ministry by focusing on purpose and passion.

- Nurture the volunteers—they need to be cared about as they go about caring for others.[13]

The third step in mobilizing volunteers is uniting. It is important for the nurse to unite the volunteers as a team. In addition to providing resources, encouragement, ownership, and affirmation of the volunteer's accomplishments, the parish nurse also can make use of buddy systems, team ministries, and mentoring opportunities that allow the volunteer to feel connected—not only to the nurse, but to the entire volunteer team as well.

In the fall of 1992, Eileen Altenhofer, parish nurse of Normandy Park Congregational Church, took a course titled Called to Care, developed by the Office for Church Life and Leadership of the United Church of Christ. The Called to Care resource notebook includes a training program aimed at enhancing the skills of laypersons interested in joining ministries of caregiving. Terry Teigen, the pastor of Eileen's church when she took this course, strongly advocated for the preparation of lay caregivers and worked with Eileen and others to develop a caregiving ministry. The Called to Care lay ministry was actually established before parish nursing was instituted. Laypersons were trained to provide support to members of the congregation during times of spiritual crisis, illness, or bereavement through the following activities: sending cards and notes; making hospital, home, or telephone visits; maintaining prayer chains; making casseroles; providing transportation to doctor's appointments; and running errands. The lay volunteers were coordinated by Eileen and Joan Wieringa, another parish nurse. Additional volunteers were recruited from the congregation as needed, and along with Pastor Terry Teigen, Eileen and Joan provided continuing education to increase the skills of the volunteers. This ministry is still operating in 2010.[14]

Terrill Stumpf, director of Chicago Lights Center for Whole Health: A Community Outreach Program at Fourth Presbyterian Church in Chicago, submitted the following story illustrative of the value of volunteers to a health ministry:

Once in the spring and once in the fall we have a community health fair on site at the church for guests of the Chicago Lights Elam Davies Social Service Center (EDSSC), serving low-income and homeless people. It just would not be possible without all the partnerships and volunteers that go into making up the whole. In a period of two-and-a-half hours some sixty-five guests participated in the health fair on Sunday, April 18, 2010. Two international visitors from Egypt were on the church campus and participated in the health fair as well.

We partner with the Northwestern University–Alliance for International Development (NU-AID) first-year medical students at the Feinberg School of Medicine. Some twenty-two medical students and staff manage our screening stations (such as glucose screening, blood pressure screening, height/weights, vision screening, and hearing screening) and our resource station (health care and social service agency referrals, health education brochures, and condoms). The NU-AID core team of four medical students provide oversight and assist where/when needed. Two physicians from the school/clinics are on site to provide assistance and back up the medical students and offer medical advice for guests in need of a higher level of care.

The NU-AID students also staff our health education discussion stations (nutrition, general well-being—each guest receives a new pair of white cotton socks—and safer sex). These are lively, ongoing discussions with demonstrations and self-learning activities in chair circles of eight. We contract with and offer stipends to two church members for our substance abuse and stress/balance (mental health) stations, due to the need for a higher-level health care provider there.

Social service center employees and volunteers staff our check-out station—all participants receive a Passport to Wellness ticket on admission and, if they participate in three screenings and three education discussions, they receive a substantial hygiene kit (made up of soap, deodorant, toothpaste, toothbrush, razor, and shampoo, put together by volunteers prior to the health fair).

Two years ago, the NU-AID medical students added a heart and breath sounds station that also requires a faculty physician consultant. Together with that, a Soul Sounds station was added. It's a creative arts expression station, staffed by two volunteers from the church. Spread out on a large table are postcard-sized pictures of nature, colored marking pens, an array of colored construction paper, and glue sticks. The fair's question in 2010 was this: What comes to mind when you hear the word *freedom*? Participants are encouraged to first select a picture(s), colored pen(s), and colored construction paper. Then they are prompted to draw, write a phrase, a sentence, a poem, and the like in response to the question. Once each creative art expression is completed, it is placed on a whiteboard, making up a collage for all to see. Participants can sign or not sign their names. Some fifty-two guests participated in spring 2010. One guest wrote, "Cloudless night/Full moon/We are free to gaze into the night sky." It never seems to fail. The volunteers are always blown away by the vulnerability and engaged stories the guests share with them, the meaningful responses, and the picture selections. Every time I go by the table, they beckon me to see one of the Soul Sounds. One volunteer commented on the experience, saying, "They gave me more than I gave to them. My soul was touched."

For this health fair, we partnered with Chicago House to provide rapid HIV/AIDS confidential testing, counseling, referrals, and case management. Bus transportation passes are provided to those who want to take advantage of the case management. To maintain confidentiality for our guests, the bus passes are given to the Chicago House staff to give out during their counseling and referral sessions.

One social service employee and two volunteers staff the check-in and registration table. If a guest is not familiar with the EDSSC, information is provided. Participants then go to one of four heart and cardiac history assessments before going into the health fair booths.

Two years ago, we had an Albert Schweitzer Fellow, one who provides two hundred hours of health care or social services to underserved and vulnerable populations. She was a graduate family nurse-practitioner student from St. Xavier University School of Nursing. She provided a health and wellness drop-in service each Sunday before the church's Sunday Evening Supper for our social service guests. Her fellowship ended, but she continues to provide such services on a volunteer basis one to two Sundays a month. She is a nurse in the cardiovascular clinic at Northwestern Memorial Hospital. But that's not the end of the story. She has worked out arrangements with a staff cardiologist, an EKG technician, and an echocardiogram technician to provide the equipment for a basic EKG and a screening echocardiogram for those guests who need further testing based on intake cardiac history, blood pressure reading, and heart/breath sounds. Seven participants needed the additional testing, following the procedures, and she provides the cardiac health education. For the three out of the seven who needed further health care, she made referrals and connections for care at the cardiology clinic. This whole additional level of care is arranged by her, and all the treating professionals are volunteers. The cardiologist sees the individual in the clinic after hours, generic prescription medications are obtained through Target's low-cost prescription plan. This nurse then contracts with the guests to be seen and followed at the health and wellness drop-in service on Sundays.

The health fair is located in two different areas in the church's basement for the screening and education stations. We used three conference room spaces on the first floor of the education building for the hearing screenings and the rapid HIV/AIDS testing for quiet and confidentiality. This necessitated a waiting area. Because of all the locations on two different levels, we had four volunteers stationed in key areas to provide hospitality and directions, and to answer questions about where particular booths were. There were three coffee stations, providing caffeinated coffee (our guests informed us via a focus group that this was an incentive and reward) and fresh bananas. A church member gives two cases of bananas as an in-kind donation. With the number of volunteers at check-in, checkout, and providing directions, we had no reports of anyone getting lost or complaints that they "couldn't find something."

All six of the spaces used for the health fair are also used for various events as part of Sunday worship and activities of the church. This means that there is a very brief window of time to transform and set up the spaces—it all has to be done within one hour. It would be overwhelming without the cooperation of the church's house staff and numerous volunteers (Loyola Academy High School community service students), who are stationed around the building. When a room is vacated, they move in and help with the transformation and setup.

There were a total of thirty-two volunteers from the church and the community providing a combined eighty hours of work and ministry. In addition, there were six staff members who provided fifteen hours of work and ministry. These numbers do not take into account the numbers and hours of the house staff, security guards, and receptionist, all on duty during the time of the community health fair—they would have been on duty anyway.

The total numbers only tell a partial story of volunteering—all the organizing, planning, recruiting, and orienting of volunteers. The human resources tell another part of the story. Each of the medical students maintains eye contact with all our guests, calls them by name, listens with spiritual intention, provides safe touch as appropriate, and speaks *with* rather than *to* our guests, as do our other volunteers from the church or community. The environment is well-organized and runs smoothly; it is festive and enjoyable. All told, there is opportunity provided for each and every guest to experience a healing environment of welcome and hospitality. Just as each guest is touched in some way in body-mind-spirit, each volunteer and staff member is touched as well. A foretaste of the Kingdom to come.

So, may it be so. Amen.

Mary Mauer, a parish nurse at St. Bartholomew Episcopal Church in Pewaukee, Wisconsin, for six years, describes the value of volunteers:

I have been a parish nurse at St. Bartholomew Episcopal Church for six years. I am passionate about my parish nurse ministry and realized early on that I am limited in the number of people to whom I personally can minister. I have been very blessed that St. Bartholomew is a training center for Community of Hope lay pastoral caregiver training. This program involves a forty-two-hour training for lay pastoral caregivers, based on Benedictine spirituality. There is a written curriculum and a faculty of speakers for each of the twelve modules. These modules focus on training lay pastoral caregivers to be a noncontrolling, listening presence. We train members from our congregation as well as parishioners from many other Christian churches in the area. This training has become so popular that we hold two classes per year.

Training volunteers is a priority for me so that I can multiply my ministry by sending out these well-trained lay pastoral caregivers to be my eyes, ears, hands, and feet. I have been a facilitator for this program since I began my parish nurse ministry as I realized how valuable well-trained volunteers can be to me, my ministry, and the church. They visit and make contacts, and then report back to me any needs or concerns they encounter.

While visiting a shut-in, one of my volunteers recognized that she was slightly confused. I was called and joined my volunteer at our parishioner's home. I knew that she had had a history of urinary tract infections, which were manifested initially by confusion. I called her doctor and scheduled an appointment for that afternoon. Her doctor started her on antibiotics. Her son stayed with her until her confusion subsided. She was able to remain in her home, as was her wish. Her doctor told us at a return appointment that had she not been seen as promptly as she was, she would have ended up in the hospital.

My well-trained lay pastoral caregiver was integral to alerting me and getting our parishioner the help she needed very promptly. I thank God for my volunteers and the ways in which they extend my ministry.

Most of the literature on parish nursing describes the value of volunteers in supporting the chronically ill elderly in their homes, but the value goes beyond this age group to encompass the needs of younger families as well. Buijs and Olson describe the use of volunteers to support young families with babysitting services as well as grocery shoppers, meal providers, and drivers. There exists the possibility of linking older parishioners who are isolated from their own families with children from other families within the church community—providing a surrogate grandparent-grandchild experience.[15]

Organizer of Support Groups
Support groups are an effective way to help individuals deal more effectively with a broad range of life stresses. From fighting an alcohol and/or substance abuse addiction to coping with the death of a young child, support groups, usually run by laypeople, offer spiritual

counsel and comfort, decrease isolation, enhance a sense of connectedness, and enable people to gain new insights and perspectives. As a result, they figure prominently in promoting health and wellness. The role of the parish nurse includes organizing and facilitating support groups, such as the Recovery from Loss group developed by Carole Kornelis, parish nurse at First Reformed Church in Lynden, Washington. This group meets for nine weeks and deals with all aspects of loss, regardless of whether the loss occurred through death, divorce, unemployment, or the ending of a relationship.[16] Other times the parish nurse's role is to disseminate information to the congregation regarding already existing community-based support groups.

Debbie White, chairperson of the Parish Health Ministry at St. Stephen Martyr Catholic Church in Louisville, Kentucky, shared the story of the church's ministry, Health of St. Stephen, or HOSS. This is a well-organized group of nurses who function as a subcommittee of the Health Ministry. Debbie says about this ministry: "The Spirit has truly been alive and guiding us and we just keep growing and touching more and more lives all through our Stewardship." One of the many activities sponsored by HOSS is an exercise–weight reduction support group modeled after the television show *The Biggest Loser.* In 2009, fifty-five individuals worked hard at this twelve-week program to try to lose weight by adopting healthy lifestyles along this way. This initial program spawned "HOSSLOSS" walkers, who meet two times a week to walk together.

Referral Agent and Liaison

The role of the parish nurse is not to replace what is already being offered within a community but to help parishioners access existing appropriate resources to meet their particular needs. In order to fulfill this role, the parish nurse must develop an in-depth knowledge of exactly what is available within the church community. For example, the church might provide volunteer services to help with specific needs, such as home visitation, a food pantry, and/or emergency funds to assist a parishioner in the short term. The nurse needs to know what is available within the surrounding community, such as flu shot clinics; free mammograms for breast cancer screening; and home health care, respite, homemaker, and transportation services. Additionally, the nurse must know how to access these resources, how these resources are paid for, whether they provide transportation, and what the waiting time is for appointments.

The nurse needs to communicate with hospital-based discharge planners, primary care physicians, specialists, clinics, and any other provider within the health delivery system. Two other health care specialists that the parish nurse must communicate with are chaplains and pastoral counselors. To some, the role of the parish nurse may seem to compete or overlap with that of chaplains and pastoral counselors. Yet, there is much more room for each to complement the others than to compete against them. The needs for spiritual care may be so enormous that spiritual resources may be stretched to their limits. The primary domain of the chaplain and the pastoral counselor is the formal health care setting (hospitals, nursing homes, outpatient clinics, etc.), whereas the primary domain of the parish nurse is the community (and, more specifically, the religious community). There is tremendous need for the spiritual care delivered in the health care setting to be continued in the patient's home, family, and religious environment. This requires close communication between chaplains and parish nurses, particularly around the time of hospital or clinic discharge, or at the time of hospital or nursing home admission. Each will find the other a tremendous resource in helping to meet the patient's or family's spiritual needs on an ongoing basis.

The nurse has a pivotal role in linking church members with these services and helping them to navigate the turbulent waters of the health care system. Marianne Parker notes the importance of parish nurses serving as liaisons not only with congregational and community resources but also with state and federal parish nurse contacts. These are essential to ensure that the nurse remains current when it come to emerging trends, regulations, and resources that directly affect the practice of parish nursing.[17]

Debbie White of St. Stephen Martyr Catholic Church shares

some wonderful stories of the role played by parish nurses in getting parishioners to the right health care professional.

One parishioner, who didn't realize he had hypertension, was monitored on a regular basis by one of our parish nurses who got him to a physician's office. Through education and support with weight-loss programs, he shared with us that after six months of working with us we have saved his life. He lost twenty-five pounds, he is eating healthy, exercising, and now is able to come off his medication. Another example was a young mother who was experiencing severe postpartum depression whom we referred for professional help. Today she is now feeling like an integral part of the parish and wants to give back to others.

Integrator of Faith and Health

Every parish nurse who participated in this book emphasized two key points: the importance of prayer at every juncture of their practice, and the need for constant awareness that faith community/parish nursing is God's work and He is in charge of every aspect of it. Many mentioned the necessity of praying for guidance when the call to parish nursing first becomes apparent; the need to pray as overtures are made to the congregation; the need to pray for acceptance by parishioners; the need to pray for wisdom as the parish nurse role is defined and communicated, and the boundaries are set; the need to pray as individual programs are developed, implemented, and evaluated; the importance of praying for God's guidance in each nurse-parishioner encounter; and the importance of prayer to make the link between faith and health for the parish community. Clearly, the centrality of God, prayer, and faith are paramount in the practices of those who have been called to parish nursing. As Cheryl Hovland, chairperson of the Parish Nurse Health Ministry at St. Stephen Martyr Catholic Church in Lexington, Kentucky, points out, "When you pray for someone, you begin to love them."

Some of the most powerful stories shared by nurses were those that involved the integration of faith and health. Debbie White, from St. Stephen Martyr Catholic Church, shares another powerful story:

Our parish nurse program is based on the premise that prayer is the most important thing we can do for the health of our community, so we have offered two prayer services and have a third planned for the fall of 2010. We started a Prayer Request Book for church that is brought to our meetings and we offer prayer for the requests written in the book. We, along with our schoolchildren, now have a beautiful prayer garden that was developed and is now maintained by the parish nurses, which offers a quiet place for everyone to reflect and pray.

After one of our prayer services, a young woman lingered on after everyone else had left. She was tearful and obviously shaken. When I approached her to see if I could help, she began hugging me and thanking me for having the prayer service. After spending some time with her, I found out that she had recently been told she had a serious health problem and had only come to the prayer service because she didn't know where else to turn. I was able to get her some resources about what was going on with her body and the disease and, with follow-up, I know that the Spirit was there at that place and in HIS time.

Health Advocate

The last function to be discussed is that of health advocate—someone who supports and defends the position of individual parishioners. In today's fast-paced and highly technological health care system, it is important for parishioners to have an advocate who will speak and stand up for their health care rights, values, and needs. It is also important for someone to affirm and validate the desires of the individual parishioner's heart. Wendy Walnock, RN, BSN, PN, parish nurse at St. Joseph's Church in Keyport, New Jersey, shares a powerful story of advocacy where she was the recipient of advocacy from the faith community that she served as a parish nurse.

Two years after beginning a health ministry at a local Catholic church (I am Methodist), I was diagnosed with breast cancer. During the first few years prior to my illness, I spent much of my time trying to educate the parishioners about parish nursing and the role of the health ministry within the confines of the church. Little did I realize that God was truly at work. After I was diagnosed, had a mastectomy, and began six months of chemo, the parishioners rallied around me with such support and faith-filled prayers that I recovered and am doing quite well. They were the ones who showed me what it really meant to be present to others, which is so much a part of being a parish nurse. This is my eleventh year at St. Joseph's Church in Keyport, New Jersey, and I feel extremely blessed that God led me here to do His work.

In summary, the parish nurse carries out an interrelated ministry of presence, word, and action to fulfill seven specific functions. These functions include acting as a health educator, a personal health counselor, a trainer of volunteers, an organizer of support groups, a referral agent and liaison with congregational and community resources, an integrator of faith and health, and a health advocate. The nurse's presence, compassion, knowledge, communication skills, and spiritual strength all combine to create a powerful ministry where the focus is more on "being with" and less on "doing for" the parishioner. The next chapter examines the soaring mountain peaks when parish nurses say, "This is why I became a nurse," and the valleys when the parish nurse feels the challenge of helping the parishioner is beyond her skill level.

3. The Journey of the Parish Nurse within the Church

Can you remember taking a trip before there were GPS systems or the detailed maps supplied by the American Automobile Association (AAA)? Going on a journey was more of an adventure when we didn't have exact directions. Life is a journey without the benefit of directional tools. It is full of twists and turns, unexpected detours, unbelievable highs and unspeakable lows. So, too, is the journey of faith community/parish nursing. And like the journey of life, the journey of faith community/parish nursing holds incredible paradoxes—joy and sorrow, happiness and grief, excitement and frustration.[1] It is never boring.

Faith community/parish nursing affords the privilege of accompanying church members as they journey through life. Sometimes the nurse is invited into the private and intimate world of parishioners. In response to this invitation, the parish nurse, acting as a facilitator, frequently transforms healing both in the individual as well as in the family. At other times, the invitation brings the nurse face-to-face with a magnitude of pain and unmet needs that not only are overwhelming but lead the nurse to question her/his ability to make a difference. The parish nurse is drawn to offer whatever is possible to ease suffering, provide reassurance, facilitate peace, bring about reconciliation, increase coping, and enhance spiritual well-being—certainly not easy tasks. However, when we asked nurses to describe the highs and lows, the joys and challenges of their journeys, the most common theme was, "Now I know why God called me to become a nurse!"

However, there were other nurses who had experienced significant pain when their efforts to develop a faith-based ministry were rebuffed or met with resistance. Some experienced unbelievable pain when, after successfully developing a spiritually rich and robust ministry, a change in ministerial leadership brought an end to their ministries. Their voices must also be heard.

Challenges of the Journey

A parish nurse-coordinator (who wishes to remain anonymous), who has worked with many faith community/parish nurses, offered the following summation of the challenges faced and endured by some of the nurses:

- Passive disinterest and nonsupport—which can suck the life out of the ministry. It potentially creates an environment where the parishioners begin to doubt the value of the ministry, because they don't hear or see the pastor supporting it.

- Triangulating with other staff, with the parish nurse/health ministry as the focus. Sometimes, though not always, this can be prompted by what is perceived to be compensation inequity. For instance, a church secretary or finance person who writes the check to a nurse, a check that is obviously bigger than what the check writer gets and perhaps is stressing the finances of the congregation, begins to make innuendos about the nurse's worth and value to the congregation. Or it can happen simply because some members of the ministry team are more tenured and "have the ear" of the pastor—and over time, the environment becomes hostile and dysfunctional.

- Inappropriate and destructive use of power against the nurse personally or the ministry in general.

- Abrupt discontinuation of the ministry with no planning for the impact on the congregation or the nurse. I have found that few pastors are well trained in human resource issues or have the skills to anticipate the impact of actions like this.

• Active undermining of the parish nursing ministry and/or taking credit for things the parish nurse accomplishes as accomplishments of the pastor. There is often little affirmation for what the parish nurse does—more often, just tolerance. This is more frequent in situations where a new pastor comes into the congregation and "inherits" the ministry. This new pastor may have no interest in learning more about the ministry (perhaps he's reluctant to admit his lack of knowledge in this area) and how it can multiply the effectiveness of his ministry. Sometimes the pastor is threatened by the nurse who has profound relationships with parishioners, so out of his limited information he "uses" the ministry and its successes to affirm himself, with a possible secondary effect of undermining the nurse and her ministry.

All of the above can happen as a result of church polity, emotionally unhealthy clergy, feeling threatened by the nurse, an inability to hear truth spoken, "inheriting" a ministry that the pastor does not support or want, and an inability to build effective relationships. These issues are apparent in the stories that follow: Parish nursing does not always have a happy ending.

Lack of Congregational Support for the Parish Nurse

When we inquired about the challenges that faith community/parish nurses faced, one of the major issues that surfaced was the issue of gaining acceptance by the ministerial staff and/or the congregants of the faith community. Sometimes this challenge was not able to be resolved and the nurse left the ministry.

Yvonne Stock approached her home church and was told that the pastor would send her an e-mail regarding his response—none was ever sent. Yvonne concluded that the Lord had something else in mind for her and she applied for and was hired as the parish nurse for CHAMPS (Center for Healthy Aging, Ministries, Programs and Services) in Omaha, Nebraska. Yvonne counsels other nurses who may be faced with resistance to parish nursing:

Always view God as the leader of the ministry and then you won't be disappointed. God's sheep bite and you might as well know that. You cannot please everyone all the time, but can love them regardless of what is occurring. Depend not on yourself, but on God—He is the King, the Comforter, and the Abba Father. Praise him when things go well and when they don't go so well. Just never stop loving people!

Lorraine Pearson was one of the nurses who shared her story of overwhelming resistance and deep pain. Lorraine served for three years at a church in Alberta, Canada, leaving to become a public health nurse. Lorraine shares:

I am sometimes sad about the time I served as a parish nurse, but now I look to how I can serve the people entrusted to me in the secular world. Funny how the people in a congregation were not interested in how I could help/serve them but people who do not know God are grateful for the care that I give. I personally had to forgive the church and its leaders for not supporting me and the vision that I was called to. It was a very long three years of trying to gain support from the pastors and the church leadership. After much prayer and tears, I left my position and our family left the church where I served. It will be coming up to three years this July and no one has called to see where I have gone. God had given me an incredible vision and I thought He would also give me some support, which was not the case. I am sure that God was trying to teach me something—I am still not sure what and why—but the experience has taught me a lot about forgiveness and letting go.

One of the saddest stories that we heard of resistance to parish nursing came from Harriet Vance who served for eleven years as a parish nurse; she requested that the location be withheld. Her ministry was rich and varied—she provided pastoral care to the elderly and homebound, including a prayer shawl ministry, a Eucharistic ministry, hospital visits, an exercise class, taking meals to a parishioner who had been hospitalized and still recovering, to name just a few. Harriet was deeply committed to health education and wrote a training program that was copyrighted. She trained teachers to follow this program; she wrote a weekly column for the church bulletin, titled "Healthy Hints by Harriet"; she provided counseling and education for parishioners and/or their children about aging and transitioning to care facilities when that was needed. She offered grief support and coordinated and trained a large cadre of volunteers. However, the ministerial leadership of the church changed and with that the culture of the church was transformed from loving and open to punitive, fearful, and closed. Harriet worked to rectify this situation. She first attempted to talk to the church leader and when that was unsuccessful went to that person's superior. The leadership closed ranks and, sadly and with great pain, Harriet had to resign. When we first talked to Harriet, her wounds were raw and she was in exquisite pain. She sent us poetry that she was writing as an outlet for her pain. See Box 3–1 for an example of Harriet's poetry.

Michalene King also shares the difficulties that arise when the pastoral leadership changes. Sometimes the ministry of faith community/parish nursing that was embraced and supported by one ministerial team is either rejected entirely or only weakly supported by the new leadership. Michalene, who serves as parish nurse-coordinator in Wintersville, Ohio, had this to say:

One of the most challenging experiences has been the change in pastors. Our new pastor is very supportive, but it took a while before we could even meet him to discuss the ministry—we were in limbo. Once we talked with him, it took several more months before we could schedule a meeting and now we are still reorganizing the ministry. I felt very helpless for months. I was still able to talk with parishioners about their health problems and we were still ministering to nursing home patients by bringing the Holy Eucharist to them, but that was the extent of our ministry.

Overlap with Pastor's Role

Sonja Simpson, RN, MSN, AHN-BC, a parish nurse in Arizona, shared that her most challenging issue involves sorting out her role from the pastor's role so they are not duplicating services or

Box 3.1.

Harriet's Sorrow: Confronting Evil
May 29, 2009

Confronting evil involved a high cost,
to my soul, spirit, and flesh,
resulting in wounds, tearing pain, and soul destruction.
The battle against darkness lingers ever near.
Intense, daily battling and inner conflict
result in heaviness that weighs my body down

Speaking the truth and living with integrity:
I thought it was the way to live, but it
led to many betrayals and misunderstandings;
ripping apart relationships that I believed were lifelong;
friends now questioning my faith, reliability, and uprightness,
turning their backs on me as if I now was the evil one

Menial daily tasks consume my limited energy
Pain and deep wounds steal liveliness and zest for life
leaving me to journey through each day slowly,
taking frequent quiet rest periods,
to find renewal and strength to plod on;
waiting for healing, pleading to God for light

Tears spill from my eyes when the despair fills my heart.
Meaninglessness, emptiness, loneliness race through my whole being
My spirit is crushed, my soul aching, my physical body now
a container for nothing but sadness and darkness
Will I ever find the light? Will I ever experience life in my being?
Will I ever feel anything but sadness?

Will God provide what is needed to restore my health?
Will He protect me from evil? Is His strength greater?
Hiding in the orchestra pit, waiting for the music to burst forth
the woman in black hides behind her dark glasses
hiding her grief, trying to find a safeguard and defense
for the cruelty of what has happened to her

Box 3.1. (cont.)

The Battle
June 4, 2009

I did not choose the battle
Rather it chose me

I, who believed I was going to end clergy abuse
now become the victim of even deeper clergy abuse

Destruction of my person is the punishment
for attempting to bring health to the church

To silence me becomes the ultimate goal;
to control my every move was their aim

Now I become the target and focus of the battle;
my soul caught between good and evil

Total collapse of my confidence,
enthusiasm, delight, and love for life

A brilliant career destroyed
as meaninglessness rules every day

A deep dark hole replaces energy and passion
leaving exhaustion and fear of evil consuming me

Betrayals are exchanged for once strong friendships;
other relationships are destroyed in the battle

Death all around and deep inside
swallowing me to the core of my being

Cold to the core like standing outside a concentration camp
in the snow without clothes—shaking in fear

My soul looks like a dull lifeless terrain:
barren, dry, and godforsaken

Box 3.1. (cont.)

An empty shell remains
An empty hollow void swallows me up

Excruciating psychic pain rules
for which there is no relief except tears

Tears, tears, and more tears
Will they ever stop?

Evil seems to steal all goodness
within me and in relationships which I loved

What will bring healing or relief—
reading scriptures, praying, playing piano?

Quiet, being alone, solitude?
Trying to do kindness for others from an empty soul?

The battle between good and evil is a lonely journey
feared by most and understood by few:

This breakdown of what makes a person human,
this injustice where there is no evidence of God's reign

Catastrophic loss of my person, relationships, successful career,
responsible work history, church and faith-life, all meaning in life

Deep despair and discouragement hang on my body
like a heavy cloak which makes life nearly impossible

What happens when one's spirit has been crushed?
Where is the light, the fire inside now contained?

Coming close to the sight of the abuse causes great anxiety within
Fear of repeated attack presses in; panic and terror smother me

What is there left to cling to? Where can I find safety?
Is anxiety the only answer to all the questions?

When will I be free to return home, to safety?
When will the battle between good and evil subside?

—Harriet Vance

competing with each other. According to Sonja, "This is a very sensitive topic, not only for me but, I think, for most parish nurses."

Lack of Involvement and Financial Support

Sharyn Farner, a parish nurse at Messiah Lutheran Church in Halifax, Pennsylvania, shares that her major challenge has been in getting people in her congregation involved in the program and in gaining adequate financial support to allow for growth, outreach, and educational programs.

For instance, I have repeatedly asked for funding for an AED (Automated External Defibrillator). This request has repeatedly been denied by both the pastor and the congregation as being unimportant, despite the fact that the majority of the congregation is older or elderly with serious health issues. I feel sometimes that instead of the health ministry team and pastor working with me and helping me, they leave me on my own to do things or just push me away. For the past two years I have organized a health fair and each year get less help and support, so much so that I have decided not to do it again.

Lack of Time

The issue of too many needs and not enough time was a frequently expressed challenge by the faith community/parish nurses. Many of the nurses who shared their stories continued in their full-time jobs while trying to balance family demands and a ministry to the church—resulting in a sense of being overwhelmed and perhaps of doing a lot of things but doing none of them well.

Dr. Emmerentia du Plessis, a parish nurse and psychiatric nurse specialist from South Africa, shares her challenge in trying to balance a full-time faculty role with the demands of her clinical specialty and the needs of her congregation.

I am employed full-time at the university, and as I am still developing as an academic and clinical specialist, I am involved in a wide variety of tasks and projects. Also, the pastor is only part-time in the congregation, and also has other academic and clinical (pastoral counseling) responsibilities.

Humbled by Another's Pain

Elizabeth Pokorny from St. Margaret Mary's Church in Council Bluffs, Iowa, shares an experience where she was participating in a blood pressure screening:

A parishioner came to our blood pressure table after one of the evening Masses. She was morbidly obese and earlier in the day she had fallen. She shared that it had been difficult for her to get up from the fall. She decided to come to our table when the priest announced that blood pressure would be checked after Mass. She moved slowly, using her walker; she staggered as she moved forward; her eyes were downcast. I wondered whether she was trying to avoid the stares of others. As I greeted her and started to converse, I had this feeling that I was there for a reason. As we talked, I learned about the fall earlier in the day. One of our retired nurses was helping me that evening and she noticed the sadness of this woman and was especially concerned about her. I asked the woman if she had seen a physician after her fall and she told me that she had gone to see a physician who told her that he could not help her because he lacked equipment large enough for her. I saw her dilemma and my heart went out to her. She continued to talk and shared how people at her workplace would watch her when she ate and she felt they were judging her based on how much she did or did not eat—as if "Who are you kidding?" was going through their minds. Thankfully, her blood pressure was only slightly elevated and she had no apparent muscle or bone injuries. I reassured her that I would find appropriate physician resources and call her with that information in the next week. My heart went out to her—she felt embarrassed about her weight and there were so few resources that I could share with her. This encounter also opened my eyes to the special needs of the morbidly obese parishioner.

Joys of the Journey

By far, nurses shared more stories of joy than challenge. The stories encompassed eight themes:

1. the importance of presence

2. facilitating family healing

3. accompanying another along a journey of pain and uncertainty

4. assisting another toward a peaceful death

5. facilitating forgiveness

6. facilitating an unexpected healing

7. making the right connections between people

8. bringing together a community of healing and love

Throughout these stories is woven the importance of spiritual care and specifically the importance of prayer.

The Importance of Presence

Jennifer Soika shared a lovely story of her two-year relationship with Rose, an eighty-five-year-old woman in very poor health, who lived alone and taught Jennie about the importance of presence:

When I first met Rose, I was new to parish nursing and was practicing in a large Catholic congregation. Rose was in the intensive care unit (ICU), frightened, alone, and confused. She thought I was her daughter when I first came to visit her. She was recovering from peripheral vascular bypass of the left leg. Apparently, she had been in and out of the hospital several times over the last year for poor circulation and infections in her left foot. The last time I would see Rose would be in that same ICU, but over the course of two years I would develop a relationship with this parishioner that embodied what it means to be a parish nurse—working with clients wholistically, addressing body, mind, and spirit.

Rose truly was alone. Her daughter and grandson lived in another state, and though they talked frequently on the phone, they rarely visited her. Her relationship with her son was strained; he lived nearby but it was his wife who was the main caregiver. I was in contact with both the son and daughter, but it was the daughter-in-law who I worked with in helping to maintain Rose's independence safely. Rose lived in her own apartment in a senior community. It was of the utmost importance to her to be able to stay in her apartment and not be a burden. But she had very little physical contact with people. Her daughter-in-law would visit at least once or twice a month. She would talk with some of her neighbors on occasion, she would talk with the pharmacy tech when her prescriptions were delivered, and her cleaning lady came twice a month.

So Rose was very grateful when I started home visits following her discharge from the hospital. Initially, I visited to check on how she was managing alone and to bring communion, as she was unable to get to church. It was soon apparent how vulnerable and frail she was. Not only did she have poor circulation in her lower extremities, but she was being treated for heart failure, osteoporosis, and depression. Shortly after the postsurgical home health care visits stopped, I became concerned about a draining incision wound. With Rose's permission, I called her primary care doctor and facilitated an appointment and follow-up. This was the first of many opportunities I had to help Rose manage her disease processes better at home. For the next two years, Rose would only be hospitalized for two short stays to treat infections in her feet. Yes, she certainly had more doctor appointments, but because she was supported and monitored closely, she was able to manage most of her infections and her heart failure at home.

But the need for more frequent doctor appointments caused another concern—transportation. Transportation is a big source of anxiety for many homebound elders. Rose tried to work her doctor appointments around her daughter-in-law's busy work schedule, which was difficult and frustrating for both of them. For grocery shopping and other errands, Rose would utilize the Regency van service or rely on helpful neighbors. I recommended and assessed Rose for Interfaith Intervention. She agreed, and we completed the application. Fortunately, due to her many needs and requests, she developed a friendship with a couple who volunteered with Interfaith and became available to respond to Rose's many needs. They made the extra effort to take Rose to all her appointments so that she didn't have different volunteers every time. When Rose became too weak to ride the shuttle or to do the shopping herself, this generous couple stepped up and did the shopping and errands for her.

Rose's frequent visits to her primary care doctor went very well. When necessary, with Rose's permission, I would call and talk with the nurse or her doctor about my concerns during my home visit. This usually helped to facilitate an appointment in a timely manner, and it gave Rose more confidence in her conversations with the doctor. She always worried that she was wasting his time, or that she really wasn't "that sick." Seeing the cardiologist by herself was another matter. She did not feel comfortable going by herself, and she was usually confused about what she was told. As her heart failure progressed and Rose struggled with more severe symptoms, her daughter-in-law made the effort to be available for those doctor appointments. A couple times it was agreed that I would meet them at the appointment. My teaching strategy for both of them concentrated on reinforcing what the doctor said; their understanding of the disease process; the importance of daily weigh-ins and record keeping; a balanced, low-sodium diet; and compliance in taking medication. On one of my home visits with Rose, she was distraught because several of her prescription medications needed to be refilled and she only had enough cash to fill half of them. The local pharmacy would deliver the medications to her door, but she would then have to pay cash. She was trying to decide between her pain medications and her new cardiac meds; and she was leaning toward the pain medication. I made a phone call to the daughter-in-law so that she was aware of the situation. She shared my concern and called the pharmacy to set up an account. Now Rose could get all her medications refilled and not worry about paying cash for them.

At one point, after monitoring her weight for so long for water gain and trying to keep it down, it was puzzling when she had unexplained weight loss. It took several attempts before Rose would admit that she just wasn't eating. She didn't have an appetite and she didn't have the energy to prepare meals, even the ready-made frozen meals that her family had prepared for her. She was feeling more depressed and lonelier. After voicing my concern about her well-being, she was more receptive when I talked to her about Meals on Wheels. The next week after our chat she had the meals delivered three times a week—a double blessing. Now she was getting nutritious meals with enough for leftovers to keep her going and she was making contact with another friendly human being. Also at this time I was contacted by the church's Boy Scout troop leader. Did I know of any elderly homebound parishioners who would enjoy being "adopted" by a Cub Scout and his family? This scout and his family brought so much joy to Rose in that last year of her life. Not only did they visit, but they would just call to say "Hi" and send her cards. And when they arranged to take her to Mass with them on Christmas day, her euphoria and gratitude filled my heart with joy.

Rose often said that her middle name should have been *worry*. She worried about everything: insurance coverage and co-pays, her independence, her failing health, her strained relationship with her son, and her relationship with God because she couldn't attend Mass regularly. As complicated as Rose's medical treatments and regimen were, what was of greatest concern for me was how to support her spiritually. I worried that I would not have the right answers or say the right things to help her. What happened over our two years together was Rose's gift to me. She reinforced for me the importance of presence. That by just being there and listening, letting her talk through her problems, I actually helped her to solve them herself. It was OK if I did not have the answers, it was OK if in my hurried day I would forget the communion host, or I would forget the scripture readings for the day. It was OK if I wasn't able to "fix" something. To be able to offer up our prayers of thanksgiving and hope together was enough.

Rose decided to have another peripheral bypass surgery. The other option was an eventual amputation of her left lower leg. And she refused. The kind of life she imagined she would lead postamputation, hobbling around on crutches or in a wheelchair, most likely in a nursing home, was not for her. She was eighty-seven years old now. She had been praying to die peacefully in her sleep, to not be a burden to anyone, and to not end up in a nursing home. She figured she would take her chances with another surgery. She did make it through the surgery, but developed complications afterwards and lingered in the ICU for two weeks. Her daughter had flown in to be with her, and when I went to visit Rose for the last time her daughter met me at the hospital. She smiled and said, "She's been asking for you."

Facilitating a Family Healing

Carole Kornelis, a parish nurse in Washington, shares a situation involving a child-parent issue:

A twelve-year-old child who attended our church was exhibiting destructive behaviors. His mother had taken him to work with her the prior day to provide some direct oversight of his behavior—but he had spent much time alone in the car. He was bored and attempted to take things apart in the car. His "mechanical efforts" ended up breaking the radio and a few other minor things. Driving home from work that day, the mother did not notice these broken items. However, the next day she again took her son to work with her and while she was driving she realized that many things were not working. She became very upset not only over the car problems but upon realizing that she would have to tell her husband, her son's stepdad, about this situation. She anticipated that her husband would become very angry with the boy—he didn't have a warm relationship with his stepson as it was. Without thinking, the mother stopped the car, ordered her son out of the car, and told him to walk the rest of the way to her workplace. She continued to drive to work. Arriving at work and realizing the foolishness of what she had done, she retraced her route, trying to find her son. When she couldn't find him, she called 911 and reported what had happened. She felt sheer panic over what might happen to her son, whom she described as very impulsive and irresponsible. Meanwhile, after the boy had gotten out of his mother's car, he had stopped at a farmhouse where he talked to the people living there. These people were mystified as to why this child was out in this rural setting all by himself. After gathering information from the boy, the child told them what church he went to, so a phone call was made to the church—where I got involved. I arranged to have him picked up—then called the mother and the police. The family was linked to social services and a family therapist. I was able to get the mother into a parenting class and her son into a social skills class. I had such a sense of satisfaction that when this boy was in need he thought of calling his church.

Accompanying Another along a Journey of Pain and Uncertainty

Many times congregational nurses are present as a church member journeys through a time of intense pain and sorrow. This is a privileged and sacred opportunity. The nurse is called to "be with" rather than to "do for" the individual. There are usually no specific skills or tricks of the nursing trade to make the situation better, to fix it, or to make the pain go away. The nurse is called on to be a witness, to be a fellow sojourner, and to support with presence, prayer, and patience. The nurse is called on to draw on personal reserves of courage while looking in the face of incredible loss, death, anguish, and grief. Words are futile; only presence is fruitful.

Vickie Morley, a faith community coordinator working out of Shenandoah University in Winchester, Virginia, shares a poignant story that she called "Faith Community Nursing Takes Courage"

I didn't know her that well. In fact, even after meeting her for the third time, I couldn't remember her name. Little did I know that God would use her to change the way I practiced my ministry of faith community nursing. I had always considered myself an expert pediatric nurse and a specialist in children's issues. I had treaded very lightly on any ministry opportunity that dealt with adults, since I had little adult nursing experience in my former nursing roles. This very beautiful and broken woman taught me a powerful spiritual lesson that has permeated not only my ministry, but my life. Neither faith community nursing nor life is meant to be practiced or lived solely by my own talents and abilities. God has called me to a ministry I am not able to do with my own power and abilities. On any given day, He calls me into situations impossible for me without God's mercy, grace, and supernatural ability.

Prior to my experience with Jenny, I had only entered into "safe" situations in my FCN practice, situations that I could control, manage, or understand with a reasonable comfort level. When I received the phone call asking me to meet her in the church office to answer some questions about her son, I wasn't apprehensive about the appointment at all. It was about her young son, or so I thought. I had no idea that she would tell me she had lost her job as a result of a severe depression that had prompted her to make several suicide attempts. She had tried everything professionals told her to do, yet she was still sick, and she was scared. She confessed that she was not seeking me out for herself; she wanted me to help her with her son. He was acting out and having tremendous behavior problems due to her emotional issues. Despite my pediatric experience, I did not have a great deal of psychiatric or behavioral experience with which to help her son. I, too, became scared.

My natural inclination was to tell her I could refer her to a good child psychologist, give her the information, pray with her, and keep her at distance. It was not my nature to get involved with situations for which I did not have "answers" or "skills," and that I could not feel secure in handling. So I did what I knew to do as a professional nurse: I suggested the name of an excellent child psychologist; she already had one. She actually didn't want a referral. I gave her information in the form of a pamphlet and a book from our church resource library on suicide from a spiritual perspective. It was "perfect" in that it offered information on how suicide attempts affect family members. She had already read many things, and was not interested in taking these materials with her. What she did allow me to do was pray with her, but confessed that was not what she wanted, either.

When I asked her what she wanted, she said she wanted me to tell her that her son would be okay if she committed suicide. After we talked, it came to me. What she thought she wanted was an escape, but God revealed to me that what she really wanted was HOPE. She felt hopeless, and she wanted someone to tell her that this would all go away and that she, her son, her husband, and her life would all be normal again. I could not tell her that because I did not know that to be true from where I sat that afternoon in my office. I was in over my head, and I knew it.

I had a very strong prayer life and I read scripture nearly every day, but until this experience, I had never really seen or felt the supernatural power of God coming in and doing for me (and her) what I could not do for myself in the way it happened for me that day. I heard words coming out of my mouth during our conversation after that prayer that did not spring from my own mind. And I was able to hold her as she sobbed. I was able to convince her lovingly to allow the pastor to become involved.

Over the next few weeks, amazing things happened. She became involved in a small women's Bible study group; her husband began meeting with the pastor weekly; her son became involved in the church children's program in a very active way; and it seemed that healing had truly occurred. When she attempted and nearly succeeded in committing suicide again, we were all devastated. I felt like a failure. Her Bible study group, the pastor, and her husband were all frustrated, scared, and wondered how they had missed the signs. Jenny was also scared, and wanted one of us to be with her every day and every evening when her husband could not be there as he worked ninety minutes away. The small group, including me, allowed her to call us at any time—day or night—and one of us was there with her at all times when her husband could not be there, thinking this is what would keep her alive. That lasted a while, until we all began to get tired, and our own families became resentful.

We all learned a great deal about suicide over the next few weeks. I made arrangements for a local expert to come in, do a debriefing, support us, and help us process this. What we were able to do as a group was to model for this couple the power of telling the truth in love, not quitting, continuing to love and care in a healthy manner, and not enable manipulative behavior. In the conference room of the church with her family (including her husband, her mother, and her sister), every member of her small group—plus her counselor, the pastor, and I—all told her how much we loved her and wanted her to live. We told her why she was important in our lives. We also told her how her behavior had affected us and our families. We told her that we could not control whether or not she committed suicide in the future, but that if she did, we would all know it was not because of a lack of our love or commitment to her. We all signed a contract that she wrote in her own handwriting in that meeting in which she promised not to harm herself. She also promised in the contract that she would call one of us if she was having suicidal thoughts again. We all signed this, cried, and prayed. The counselor wanted to call this a contract; our pastor suggested we call it a covenant. It worked.

The counselor helped us understand that although we could not control this young woman, we could love her. Sometimes that is all that is needed to heal—the courage to love and hope. There were no guarantees, however. She made it clear to us that Jenny might still commit suicide. It was not about how much we loved or did not love her; our love could not keep her alive. We learned that the root word of both the words *encourage* and *discourage* is *courage*. We all had to have the courage to love and support her despite the potential outcome. We had to leave the result to God. We could not be God for her. We could only point her toward Him. Our being available to her 24/7 allowed no room for God. We had become God in her life. She didn't "need" God; she had us.

For me, I saw the body of Christ come alive and support this young family back to health. I saw true collaboration with professionals from our local mental health community. I saw God doing for me, our church, and this family what we could not do for ourselves. This experience changed the way I practice faith community nursing. Now I know that I do not have what it takes to be a faith community nurse; but thank goodness, God does. I am too weak, but He is strong. I am without answers to many questions, but He is the God of knowledge, wisdom, and power.

I learned that as faith community nurses, God has not called us to do what we are able to do. He calls us to do what we are unable to do *without His help*. He calls us to see the invisible, and to do the impossible. If we are able to do it, then we often become prideful and self-sufficient, and do not lean on Him. There is no "security" in what we are doing . . . only in Who God is. Only when trusting in the nature, goodness, and provision of God will we be able to sustain a practice of faith community nursing over the long haul, which is truly healing for us and for those whose lives we are privileged to touch. However, we will only do these things if we are secure in the nature of God, not ourselves.

"Nevertheless, Do not fear. I am with you." This is His answer to human weakness. He is the great God who sends us out as lambs among wolves. Why? Because the Lion is walking beside us.

How do we do this? We do it afraid. May our fear of missing God and His calling for us exceed our fear of doing what He has made us and called us to do. And when we feel discouragement, may we remember that *courage* is the root of that word, and ask God to transform it to encouragement.

Assisting Another Toward a Peaceful Death

Ruth Syre, MSN, RN, FCN, congregational health program coordinator for the Department of Pastoral Care, Centra, in Lynchburg, Virginia, tells a touching story of how she helped a dying woman and her family accept death:

Mrs. J. had been diagnosed with advanced cancer, and opted to not pursue any aggressive treatment. A widow, she lived alone in an apartment, but a supportive family was nearby. Early on, I asked if it was all right to broach some subjects that are hard to think about. She was very open, and seemed to welcome discussions about end-of-life issues. She was very much at peace, and not concerned about the inevitable decline of her health. I asked her what her plans were when she could no longer care for herself and live alone. She replied that she would move into hospice. While we do have a residential hospice facility, beds are limited, and patients must be enrolled in the hospice program with time to process such a placement. So I told her that it wasn't that simple, but I would do my best to make sure that hospice was called and she was cared for. The pastor was aware of our plan, and we occasionally coordinated joint visits in order to share the sacrament of holy communion with her. Months went by and she did relatively well, declining slowly. One day, the pastor called me from her home, saying, "It's time. Something has to be done." I immediately completed the hospice referral, and the admitting nurse visited the next day. Mrs. J never made it to the hospice facility. She didn't need to. With the support of the hospice team, her family was able to provide all the care she needed in her own home, and she died peacefully, surrounded by those she loved. I know that my asking the tough questions early on paved the way for a peaceful transition for Mrs. J and her family at her life's end.

Facilitating Forgiveness

Donna Kremer, a minister and the coordinator of congregational health for WellStar, shares her story of dealing with a forgiveness issue.

A member of our church was slowly dying of prostate cancer. For several months he attended our church's monthly Service for Healing and Wholeness. We laid hands upon him, prayed, and anointed him with holy oil. When he died, a woman angrily confronted me with the utter futility of this practice. Her friend was not cured; therefore the Healing Service was bogus in her mind. We talked at length about the concepts of healing and cure and how one could be healthy despite a terminal diagnosis (and vice versa). This led to her disclosing a grudge she had continued to harbor for more than twenty-five years. We talked of the physical and spiritual fallout she had experienced over all those years and then we prayed—for forgiveness, healing the wounds, and peace. Forgiveness has been a slow process for her, but we continue to enter the churning waters together, confident of God's healing presence.

Interpreting the difference between *healing* and *cure* continues to be a challenge. Meeting people where they are, on their own theological playing field, requires much more listening and tongue-holding than I would have ever imagined.

Facilitating an Unexpected Healing

Terrill Stumpf relates a story from his days as a parish nurse in San Francisco:

I was a parish nurse at Old First Presbyterian Church and working one day a week at the Seniors Activity Center—I had open office hours every Monday. One of the former members of the center (an eighty-year-old woman) had recently moved out of state and she was back in San Francisco on vacation. She stopped by the center to see me. We were having a friendly chat and catching up when she started to tell me that she had been depressed and was taking an antidepressant medication. She had questions about the medication. So I looked up the medication in a drug reference book. I checked indications, side effects, etc., and I shared this information in terms she could understand. As I was reviewing precautions for taking this medication, I pulled my glasses down on my nose (this was before I admitted to needing bifocals) and said teasingly that she shouldn't take this medication if she was pregnant. She looked at me, her face clouded over, and her eyes began to tear. I asked a probing question about the meaning of her tears and she began to relate a story of pain, guilt, and betrayal.

When she was twenty years old she had a relationship with a man who forced her to engage in sex. This happened again with a different young man when she was twenty-five years old. Both of these encounters resulted in pregnancy. Both times she was forced to move away from her hometown because of the shame of being pregnant and unmarried. She carried two daughters to term and then gave both of them up for adoption. For the last sixty years she had carried enormous guilt not only for becoming pregnant outside of marriage but also for giving up her children. She told me that because of the stigma, her sense of sinfulness, and the intense guilt that she felt, she had never shared her story with anyone, including her pastors. When she moved out of San Francisco, she tried to locate her two daughters. She discovered that they were both living in the state where she had relocated. She contacted them separately, and she received very warm receptions from both daughters. As she was telling me this part of the story, her face glowed with a sense of peace. I was struck by the fact that even though she had carried this guilt for all these years, in reconnecting with her daughters she had achieved a degree of peace that could carry her through the remaining years of her life. I told her that I believed that God had really gifted her with His grace and that this grace must provide some sense of relief for her guilt. With that we both started crying.

Often I think that parish nurses get so caught up in our tasks that we miss opportunities to open windows to spiritual healing. I wonder if I had not used a bit of humor, regarding her need to be cautious about pregnancy, if I would have been able to open the window that allowed her to express her guilt and sorrow. After all these years, she still carried guilt about giving up her daughters, about getting pregnant when she wasn't married, about feeling angry and betrayed at the hands of two men who had taken advantage of her. As a nurse, one part of me felt that I should explore other parts of her story—like how she had handled this situation with her own parents and how these situations had affected her decision never to get married—but I decided to just let her lead the conversation and share what she wanted to share. We ended up praying before she left and we said that we would see each other in church that Sunday. Sadly, I didn't see her Sunday and we never saw each other again. When she left, she had a glow on her face and I said, "Let the healing begin." As I reflected on this encounter, I felt that we had shared sacred space; I felt both humbled and at the same time very honored that she had shared this information with me.

Making the Right Connections between People

Because it is impossible for the parish nurse to be the only one who can make situations better, it is essential that the nurse become a multiplier of people and resources. Just as it is important for the nurse to assess what is needed in a given situation, it is just as important for the nurse to make the right connections between and among people so that healing occurs.

Anna Friedberg, coordinator of the health ministry team at a small church in East Syracuse, New York, shares an example of being a good "matchmaker":

I will never forget when one of our church members was ill and unable to manage the housework. I knew of another church member who is learning disabled but is certainly able to do housework. I paired them up and it turned out even better than I anticipated. I only thought that I was getting housework done for the one woman, but I guess God had other plans. The woman who was ill was assisted with her housework. However, the learning disabled woman loved to hear Bible stories read out loud so the woman who was ill read scripture and helped the learning disabled woman with her reading skills as well!

Bringing Together a Community of Healing and Love

The last story of joy is shared by Kristine Holmes, RN, BS, a parish nurse at First Presbyterian Church of Howard County in Columbia, Maryland. She describes how a community came together for healing and love.

Chapter 3

In the summer of 2000 a young couple returned to our church family after a brief time away. The wife informed me that after experiencing numerous miscarriages she was finally pregnant. Later in the month she told me that they were expecting triplets. We discussed resources available to them, including their own family, the church family, and organizations such as Moms of Multiples. I agreed to check her blood pressure each week, as directed by her physician.

In early September she developed hypertension and was placed on bed rest. I coordinated a meeting of the Health Ministry Team, deacons, and women's associations to develop a plan to assist her with meals and friendly visits. I continued to visit frequently to monitor her blood pressure. The members of the church's Prayer Tree lifted mom and babies up in prayer. In late October she went into labor and was admitted to the hospital.

On November 3, Charlie, Carrie, and Katie were born by Cesarean section and each weighed in at slightly over two pounds (1 kg). The congregation prayed mightily for these babies and their parents. Word spread to other congregations in the area as well as out of state, and more prayers were offered for their health and safety.

Our associate pastor and I were allowed to visit the Neonatal Intensive Care Unit regularly. We prayed with the parents and with the hospital staff. I brought pictures of the babies to the church and placed them in my office window. This eventually became a visual growth chart that I updated with new pictures after every hospital visit. Members of the congregation made a point to walk by my office so they could check on the babies. We provided regular progress reports to the congregation during our church services and to the members of the Prayer Tree.

During one of my visits to an elderly (eighty-six-year-old) homebound woman, I told her about Charlie, Carrie, and Katie. She eagerly said that she would pray for them. Part of my weekly duties then included a phone call or visit to update her on the progress of the babies. She became their "prayer warrior."

Just before Christmas, Charlie came home. The deacons and women's association continued to provide meals and assistance so that Mom could visit Carrie and Katie, who remained in the hospital. Carrie came home in early January and Katie, whose stay was lengthened because of two surgeries, was able to come home at the end of January, on Super Bowl Sunday. How appropriate that the Baltimore Ravens won the game! Once again, I took a photo—this time with a Ravens blanket covering their car seats. "Moms" of all ages pitched in to fold clothes, rock babies, wash dishes, and prepare meals. The babies' eighty-six-year-old prayer warrior continued to pray.

On Mother's Day, at six months of age, the triplets were baptized. I was privileged to assist during the service and I carried Charlie down the aisle to introduce him to his church family. As the pastor, a deacon, and I carried the children, members of the congregation reached out to touch them, as if to touch God's special work.

Two weeks after their baptism, I helped Mom load the babies into their van and we took them to see their prayer warrior—a wonderful woman who had faithfully held them in prayer. What a wonderful sight! Smiling babies and a woman whose heart overflowed with joy. *Those* pictures are in frames in my office.

Prayers, love, the helping hands of young and old, an entire community, helped strengthen this young family and our whole congregation. I am humbled to have witnessed God's abundant grace.

As we have listened to the stories of parish nurses, we hear them tell us that faith community/parish nursing involves a call, a response of faith to that call, and an unending journey. Throughout the journey we hear the voices of nurses sharing stories of challenge and joy that, woven together, form a tapestry of love, service, and dedication. In a very real sense, the journey is the destiny. In the next chapter we hear those voices sharing how God has taken their journey beyond the church and into the community at large.

4. The Journey into the Community

Journeys have a way of producing detours and side trips that are not part of the original itinerary. Most of us map out our path by identifying the most direct route and trying to avoid detours that add time or hazards to the trip. Our goal is to reach our destination. However, if indeed the journey is the destination, we may find unexpected joys when we wander off the beaten path, especially when those meanderings are not part of our planned agenda.

Most nurses involved in faith community/parish nursing plan a journey that focuses their energies on the needs of a specific congregation. As with any journey, a traveler needs to plan ahead. The traveler needs to know what to pack; she needs to know the terrain; she needs to know what personal resources are required; and she needs to know the expected time of arrival. As nurses reflect on whether or not they are called to faith community/parish nursing, they embark on a similar process of preparation. They pack their nursing knowledge and skills, along with a deep commitment that they are responding to God's call. They take stock of the "lay of the land" of their own congregation, deciding whether the territory is friendly or hostile toward a health ministry. Beyond their nursing expertise, they reflect on the personal resources that are required, such as infinite patience, excellent communication and negotiation skills, the ability to work with groups, knowledge of scripture and the faith statements of their own denomination, and the ability to draw out the best from others. They engage in additional preparation for the journey through their reading about this nursing specialty and their enrollment in various faith community/parish nursing preparation courses. They are usually confident about where they are going on this journey, although they generally underestimate the time required to arrive at a destination point where faith community/parish nursing is firmly established in their congregation. These nurses are sometimes surprised to discover that God has other plans and the destination to which He calls them is beyond the walls of the congregation!

In many places in scripture we read about journeys that took unexpected twists and turns. In the Hebrew scriptures we read how God led the Israelites out of the familiar land of Egypt and allowed them to wander through the Sinai desert, experiencing years of adventures, close calls, and unexpected opportunities. In the same way, He leads nurses from the familiar territory of hospital- or community-based nursing into the new and uncharted land of congregational nursing and beyond that to the role of educator for parish nurses, coordinator for networks of congregational health ministries, as well as to an unmapped frontier of faith-based community nursing.

These forays beyond the individual church and into the community are an extension of what God calls nurses to do within the church—educate the unlearned, support those who are unsure, calm the anxious, feed the hungry, give drink to the thirsty, clothe the naked, house the homeless, provide rest to the weary, visit the lonely, care for the sick, and offer employment to the jobless. These needs exist in our churches, our neighborhoods, our cities, our country, and our world. The call of God is to take what He gives to us and, just as Jesus multiplied the fish and loaves to feed the five thousand, nurses are to multiply their individual resources to minister within churches and beyond. How has God called parish nurses beyond the confines of their churches?

In this chapter we hear a number of stories. The first story chronicles how God called Ruth Syre to minister to other parish nurses. The second story, from Wanda Alexander, a true "network builder," focuses on God's call to bring individual parish nurses into networks where, collectively, the resources for education, program development, research, grant writing, and support are multiplied by the number of parish nurses who possess a multitude of gifts and talents—the whole is greater than the sum of its parts! The third story, from Dr. Ruth Stoll, relates how God called her to develop lay ministers and to extend her faith community/parish nursing into a community-based clinic to serve some of the poorest and neediest among His kingdom. The fourth story, from Dr. Linda Witmer, describes a journey to minister to an immigrant population. In the fifth and sixth stories, we hear Kristine Holmes and Terrill Stumpf in their efforts to minister to those who are abused and wounded. The last story, told by Dr. Karen Hahn, relates how Shirley Branch was able to bring hope to the Greater Fifth Ward. Again, let's hear their voices.

A Journey of Ministry to Parish Nurses

Ruth Syre is the congregational health coordinator within the Pastoral Care Department of a local hospital system in Lynchburg, Virginia. Let's listen to her story:

I have a unique opportunity of wearing two hats in parish nurse ministry. The first, in my local congregation, is strictly voluntary. The second, in my role as congregational health coordinator, is a full-time, salaried position within the Pastoral Care Department of the local hospital system. One of the joys I have in this job is being a parish nurse to the parish nurses in the area. One of the most fun things about being the congregational health coordinator has been to witness the hand of God nudging a nurse. It is a powerful thing to see the idea take hold, the wrestling that sometimes ensues, the fear of the unknown that overwhelms, and the joy that comes with surrender to the call. My advice is that the sense of call must be there. If it is just the pastor's idea, it won't work. I also think one needs a strong sense of self and the ability to set boundaries. While the concept may tickle the young mother with several children, it may not be the right time. In small congregations, where a few people wear many "hats," adding the hat of parish nurse may not be helpful if it is just one more thing on the list of things to do.

While I do not think that seminary or CPE are prerequisites, I think the person must have a solid faith—not a stubborn faith, but a solid grounding in her faith—in order to meet people where they are in their faith journey. Nurses are doers and fixers, and we cannot fix faith journeys for others. A nurse needs to understand what it means to be a companion on the journey.

Let me share one memory I have that illustrates my role. The voice on the phone sounded a little frantic. "I have a complaint. My pastor gave me some information about a program you are offering and said I should go. I can't go. Why doesn't my pastor understand?" Susan, the parish nurse on the phone, said all that without taking a breath. She then went on to share that she had experienced a death in her family and other family members were ill and facing crises. I told her that it is okay to say no to this particular program and to anything else right now. When I asked her if she needed a parish nurse herself, she became very quiet. We talked about the need to care for self when weathering multiple personal crises, the struggles with competing expectations from workplace and church, and the desire to be able to do more. I hope I gave her just a moment when she could step back from the intensity of her situation and see God at work in her life, and help her remember that she does not have to do it all.

Being a parish nurse to parish nurses is an extremely rewarding part of my role as congregational health coordinator. Nursing, by nature, is not done in isolation. We usually begin our career working as part of a team on a unit. While our individual practice is autonomous, we usually seek out colleagues to help support what we do. In many settings parish nurses function in a solo capacity in their faith community. They may be the only health professional and/or the only "nonclergy" person on the ministerial team.

My role of support has at least two main components. The first is to be a resource and support person. I refer to my role as "chief cheerleader" for the parish nurses and health ministry teams. I am an encourager and a connector. I am also a safe place. Parish nurses can share their joys and struggles with me without worrying that it will impact their ministry. I have prayed with and for them, and they for me. The second main component is that of networker. By being at the "hub" of the wheel of health ministry in the area, I have a good sense of what activities are taking place. I can help parish nurses save time and energy by helping them locate resources for individual as well as congregational needs. I can also bring parish nurses together. When we come together we can readily identify resources that may be shared, but, just as important, we can learn from each other.

A good illustration of this is our walking programs. I began a simple walking program in my church, where members completed individual tallies of walking or related exercise. The cumulative miles were then plotted on a large map as we "walked" to Jerusalem. This was not a new concept, and I borrowed ideas from other health ministry programs around the country. Other churches within our congregational health partnership took the idea and made it their own. One "walked" across America, having virtual stops at selected cities, where they had a meal of food made famous in that city, learned about the city, and prayed for a sister church in each locale. They completed their walk with a luau, complete with the pastor playing his ukulele. Another parish nurse developed a photo gallery depicting all the places the group would "travel" in their walk to Jerusalem. Another is "walking" to all the places where they have missionaries. Each faith community takes the original idea and personalizes it to match the interest of its congregation. This is certainly evidence that we are so much better together than alone.

Nurses are also teachers, and parish nurses are no exception. While no area parish nurses are employed by our program, I serve as a support for new parish nurses. For those who complete a basic preparation course, or who have had prior experience, I may just orient them to the existence of our program and available resources. For inexperienced parish nurses, I am available to help define and implement the role. I often connect a new parish nurse with an experienced one, creating a natural mentoring relationship. With three nursing education programs in close proximity, there are increasing requests to place nursing students with parish nurses. This has worked well, and has been a mutually beneficial experience. As an older nurse, I am very intentional about sowing seeds for the future, planning for sustainability and longevity of the role.

I am blessed to have my job. I am blessed to have a wonderful boss. I am blessed to be with so many wonderful nurses and others who have answered God's call to serve here and now. I look forward to the future, knowing that God will continue to equip those who are called.

Journey to Multiply and Expand Faith Community/Parish Nursing: The Network Builder

This next story from Wanda Alexander brings to mind the scripture passage that appears in the gospel writings of Matthew 13:31–32.[1]

The kingdom of heaven is like a mustard seed which a man took and sowed in his field; which indeed is the least of all the seeds, but when it has grown it is the greatest of herbs and becomes a tree, so that the birds of the air come and nest in its branches.

God's word works in our hearts and causes a transformation from within. Just as the tiny mustard seed literally grew to be a tree that attracted numerous birds because they loved the little black mustard seeds the tree produced, God's kingdom works in a similar fashion and transforms from within the hearts of those who are open to God's leading. Wanda's heart was certainly open!

When Wanda's story began, she was not practicing as a parish nurse but as a "dyed in the wool" public health nurse. Over time her role as a community health supervisor in Minneapolis–St. Paul morphed into the coordinator of faith community nurse initiative. Let's listen to Wanda's words as she describes her journey.

I was working in a small, specialized Community Resources area of our large urban Health and Human Services Department about seven years ago when I first encountered parish nursing. I was trying to find new ways to link and provide health and human services in community-based settings and a block nurse referred me to a parish nurse. I remember feeling somewhat anxious about visiting my first church as a government employee. I was reared in that church and am a Christian, but I certainly had no planned agenda when I made this first visit. Now I'm very comfortable with government and faith community partnerships, but at that point I was rather unsure about the connection. I asked this nurse about her congregation, her role, if she knew of other parish nurses whose names she could share, and if she thought there might be a role for Hennepin County to play in facilitating the work of parish nurses. I also asked what assistance the county might be able to offer.

Six months later, I had called on more than sixty parish nurses and all the hospitals, health systems, and schools of nursing that had been involved in supporting or educating parish nurses over the past twenty years in the Twin Cities. Initially, most parish nurses thought there were between 50 and 75 parish nurses in the metro area; in 2003, by compiling everyone's lists, I was able to identify 167 active parish nursing programs in Christian congregations in the eleven-county area. I had more than 250 parish nurses on my new mailing list. Today, there are nearly 240 active programs in Christian, Jewish, and Muslim congregations, and I have more than 400 faith community nurses on the Faith Community Nurse Network mailing list.

The nurses had told me they wanted the county's help with professional education, communications and networking, and funding for new projects and programs. So I called together some of the parish nurses I'd met from various faith traditions and together we formed a nonprofit agency, the Faith Community Nurse Network of the Greater Twin Cities, to champion faith community nursing in our area. First, we began offering continuing education workshops, free of charge. Seventeen nurses attended our first workshop on Economic Assistance for Low-Income Clients, and we were thrilled. Since 2004 we have offered four workshops annually, each worth 3.6 CEUs. Our average attendance has increased every year to over ninety faith community nurses in 2009. We also get sponsors who provide box lunches, and that adds a nice time for networking after the event.

We've been very fortunate in our partnerships with other agencies. We've been able to partner with the state and county to award computers and laptops to more than fifty faith community nurses. We started a Faith Community Nursing Collection in the Hennepin County Library system of more than seventy items, all of which are available to parish nurses throughout the state. We've secured grants to enable us to award $1,000 mental health grants to thirty-nine innovative faith community nursing programs over the past few years. We've participated in some research projects and, last year, appointed a Research and Advisory Council made up of twelve leading faculty from seven schools of nursing. This year, we secured funding from our local United Way for a long-term project aimed at supporting frail elderly and their caregivers with faith community nursing resources. We also began offering Basic Preparation for Faith Community Nursing courses, led by an interfaith group of experienced local faith community nurses.

As an organization, we've been very busy. But this has been a journey of faith and renewal and revelation. I have been incredibly blessed with all the people I've met in this process. Early on I met Laura Rydholm, a brilliant angel of a woman who started the parish nursing program at Immanuel St. Joseph in Mankato, Minnesota. The first time we met, I told her my story and I also found myself sharing some concerns about potential conflicts. Laura said firmly, "Wanda, you know this is a call, don't you? You go ahead and do this work and don't let anybody stop you. You are where you are supposed to be." Laura told me that my contacts with parish nurses were like "finding gold."

Many people are very surprised that a local government would be involved with faith community nursing. I wonder why other areas of government are not. For one thing, government should support the volunteer efforts of its citizens. In the Twin Cities, faith community nurses, who are unpaid staff, contribute more than $2.6 million in services each year. Faith community nurses in the Twin Cities made more than 100,000 individual and home visits in 2009. As a professional group, we need to work on documenting the effectiveness of our efforts. A research study led by Laura Rydholm[2] (the first one in which FCNN nurses participated; Laura has written several research articles dealing with the effectiveness of parish nursing) found that one thousand interventions by faith community nurses with seniors resulted in cost savings of more than $3.25 million—in addition to countless health benefits.

Recently, I was able to have a survey commissioned with Dr. Barbara Leonard from the School of Nursing at the University of Minnesota.[3] The aim of the survey was to put together a resource and research council and to answer certain questions, including the following:

- What is the best way to prepare faith community nurses?
- How does the faith community specialty embrace and invite the nurse?

We received a 74 percent return rate on the survey; 15 percent of the nurses had master's degrees; 61 percent were BSNs. The survey gave us a better idea about the market for FCNs. One of the significant findings of this survey was that, in Hennepin County, 65 percent of all citizens and 89 percent of all seniors identify themselves as members of a faith community. So it is only logical—especially if we want to reach seniors in a group—to try to reach them via their congregations. And we all know that no professional is more trusted than a nurse.

Please take a look at our website—www.FCNNTC.org. There is a video streaming on the website that features my patient, Bill, and an amazing FCN, Valborg Tallesfrud, an eighty-four-year-old nurse and retired faculty member from St. Olaf's College. As soon as she retired thirteen years ago, Valborg took a parish nurse preparation course, started the ELCA (Evangelical Lutheran Church of America) Parish Nurse Association, and has been ministering sixty hours a week as an FCN/PN ever since!

During the first year or so of this work, I always felt I was on shaky ground. God blessed me with the best boss, Bob Olander, who believes so strongly in faith community nursing that he even joined our FCNN Board after he retired! He's a gifted man of faith, a real leader. We've been surrounded by leaders and such gifted, compassionate nurses. It's a privilege to work with such people. I thank God every day for calling me here. This is such an exciting ministry for me, and I think we are only just beginning!

I could talk forever about faith community nursing! I see it as the fulfillment of public health nursing, where we as nurses have reclaimed our historic role and are actually practicing wholistic nursing care.

Journey to Develop Lay Ministry Programs

Ruth Stoll's journey has taken her through many roles within parish nursing. She began as a teacher of parish nursing in the early 1990s and then moved into a paid parish nurse position in her own church. Later, after retiring from teaching, she assumed a part-time paid parish nurse position at St. Stephen's Episcopal Cathedral in Harrisburg, Pennsylvania. Her journey continued leading her into the development of lay ministry programs within African American churches. This is her story.

I was working as a parish nurse at St. Stephen's Episcopal Cathedral in Harrisburg, Pennsylvania. After four years, the role had been fully accepted and established within the congregation, and I felt the Lord leading me beyond St. Stephen's. Initially, I was drawn to an outreach ministry that St. Stephen's already had in place at the Children's Check-up Center (CCC). The CCC was located in a public housing complex, Hall Manor, that included five hundred apartments. Although there was an outreach to the children residing in Hall Manor, there was nothing comparable for the adults—many of them single mothers. The Executive Director of CCC was favorably inclined to the suggestion of conducting a door-to-door survey of the residents (primarily of African American and Latino descent) of Hall Manor. St. Stephen's also was supportive of this endeavor. An outreach worker of Latino descent and I offered free blood pressure screenings and administered a questionnaire to determine health risks and need in the adult residences, whether or not these people attended church, and if there was anything other than worship that their churches offered. We discovered that most of the residents didn't attend church with any regularity or at all, and their churches, for the most part, offered little beyond worship and church school. We also discovered many "storefront" churches in the area. Neither these small ethnic churches nor the larger, more established denominations were reaching significantly into this community. Only one church, a Roman Catholic church, was available with a multiple resources outreach. Health ministry was nonexistent; few of these churches had members who were health professionals.

As I became aware of the vast unmet spiritual, physical, and emotional needs, I felt God calling me to do something about it. I resigned my position as part-time parish nurse at St. Stephen's and committed myself to the development of lay models of health ministry within the African American and Latino congregations. Initially, I made some overtures to

89

the Latino churches in the area but found no receptivity at that time. I started to focus my attention on the African American churches. I met a young African American man in the legal aid society in Harrisburg who helped me make contact with three African American congregations. He suggested that I needed to come to the churches with something concrete to offer them. The Penn State Extension Agency listed and accepted my proposal for a 22.5-hour certificate program designed to develop lay health facilitators prepared to start health ministries within African American churches. Initially, my efforts focused on the three congregations where I had already made contact with the pastors and leaders. The program that I presented covered five major topics: 1) healthy lifestyles, including diet and exercise; 2) high-risk concerns of the population—including training the participants to take blood pressures readings on themselves and others; 3) preventing diabetes and dealing with complications; 4) depression and anxiety; and 5) how to use this information to start a health ministry within the congregation. These topics were covered in nine classes. In one church, eight participants completed the entire program and earned the certificate. Twice that number attended individual classes but chose not to complete the entire program. Similar results occurred in the other churches. Six completed the program in a second church and seven in the third and last church. I also offered CPR certification and two churches took advantage of this opportunity. An additional session dealt with advance health directives, and one church participated. All of the classes integrated a strong spiritual and scriptural component.

To get a program in one of the churches up and running financially, I wrote a grant proposal and submitted it to the Central Pennsylvania Episcopal Diocese; I received a $2,000 grant that came with a promise of another $1,000 if we could obtain a matching grant—which we did.

Although we considered the health facilitator role in all three churches, only two pursued its development. I accepted a position as parish nurse coordinator in one of these churches and held this position for six years. Today, both churches continue a limited health ministry primarily led by lay persons. They primarily focus on blood pressure screening and health care advocacy and referral. Even though I have left the position of parish nurse coordinator, I am still being utilized as a resource/advocate person. I find this ongoing, trusting, and supportive relationship very significant both for the congregational members and myself. It is evident in my communication with these parishioners that, for some, there continues to be growth in their health knowledge and health practices

In 2007, Dr. Stoll took a position as a coordinator of Congregational Ministry of Healing and Wholeness at the Samaritan Counseling Center in Lancaster, Pennsylvania. The center had received a two-year grant to support and expand the health ministry–parish nurse experience within Lancaster County. This was a completely new endeavor for the counseling center. Through such activities as monthly continuing education seminars, annual conferences, consultation-education training opportunities offered to churches, and a continuing of the Parish Nurse Basic Certificate Course, the concept and practice of health ministry and parish nursing has expanded and flourished, not only in Lancaster County but in southeastern Pennsylvania. The outreach efforts have included not only parish nurses but congregational care coordinators, Stephen Ministers, lay congregational caring persons, and pastors—many who provide congregational care in diverse capacities. Faculty in two local colleges with RN-BSN programs have been excellent sources of referral of nurses interested in parish nursing.

My involvement in health ministry and parish nursing continues to expand like a pebble thrown into a huge pool of water—including individuals, congregations, networking groups, and lay ministries and care coordinators/Stephen Ministers. It continues to expand from my own congregation to a regional outreach serving multiple denominations and groups. Christ's command and fulfillment is wonderfully evident to me: "God authorized and commanded me to commission you: Go out and train everyone you meet; far and near, in this way of life . . . then instruct them in the practice of all I have commanded you. I will be with you as you do this, day after day, right up to the end of the age."

Journey to Minister to an Immigrant Population

Linda Witmer, RN, MPH, MSPH, MDiv, administrative director of the RN to BS Degree in Nursing Program and associate professor of nursing at Eastern Mennonite University in Lancaster, Pennsylvania, shared the following story about moving out into the neighborhood to serve in the name of Christ:

When Pastor Janet Breneman arrived at Laurel Street Mennonite Church nearly five years ago, she urged us to extend the mission and vision of the church beyond our four walls.

Our first priority was to identify the needs in the neighborhood and partner with our neighbors to meet those needs. We defined our neighborhood as the area covered by the two blocks in each direction around the church building, which included 509 households.

Next, we developed a survey tool to guide interviews with our neighbors. We asked about the strengths and weaknesses of the neighborhood and what unmet needs there were in the household, such as food, health, dental, and clothing, and what family issues they faced, including domestic violence. Other questions focused on educational needs, such as English as a second language, nutrition, exercise, parenting, and counseling.

We informed the neighborhood and city officials of our intentions through radio, fliers, and newspaper stories. Several people in the congregation mapped out the houses, our pastor trained the interviewers, and we went out in pairs. Our goal was to involve as many people from the congregation as possible. Those who could not walk the streets prayed for the interviews and helped to process the completed questionnaires. The interviewers found great joy in meeting our neighbors.

We conducted interviews in June and July 2005. A computer expert in the congregation tabulated the results and we presented the information to the neighborhood at a community meeting. Community officials and social service agencies listened and contributed to the discussion as everyone present worked together to set priorities.

We joined our neighbors in gathering signatures on a petition asking the city to put up a stop sign and to remove a bar. We offered parenting, budgeting, and exercise classes. Keeping children and youth off the streets and preventing gang activity was of the utmost concern to parents. We responded with an annual weeklong day camp in collaboration with neighboring Alpha and Omega Church of the Brethren (a Latino congregation) and Gretna Glen Camp, a Christian camp. The Outreach Committee received a Weed and Seed grant and followed through with an intergenerational mosaic project modeled after the youth's version of the Peaceable Kingdom by Edward Hicks.

Four or five community events are planned by the Outreach Committee each year. Recent examples include our Strawberry Fest, Fall Fest, Women's Tea, Christmas program, multicultural night, concerts in the parking lot, and health fair. Church involvement on local neighborhood committees is also a priority so we can keep abreast of the issues. Our congregation is renovating a nearby house, which is being used for youth and neighborhood events.

Since the survey, we have had much involvement in the community. Outreach can be a slow process and not all activities are successful. But even if only a few people visit the church each year because of our efforts, the activities are worthwhile. Our church attendance has doubled, we have baptized new members from the neighborhood, and we are now holding bilingual services. We have learned that each new person brings a gift to be shared from which we all benefit. God has indeed been gracious to us.

Journeys to Minister to the Abused and Wounded

Kristine Holmes is active as a full-time parish nurse for First Presbyterian Church of Howard County, Maryland. However, in the last few years the Lord has extended her journey as well. Although her focus remains her congregation, she has reached out to embrace the surrounding community in several ways. Let's hear her explain.

When I began to make our congregation aware of the extent of domestic violence in the area and our responsibility as a caring community, I began by educating the congregation. I had the full support of the pastor and associate pastor as well as the health ministry team. I placed information posters in each stall of the women's restroom. The information posters included tearoff sheets on what steps to take in leaving an abuser, what precautions to take, what numbers to call, etc. Within a few days of my posting this information, every tearoff sheet was gone! Needless to say, I was surprised. I couldn't believe—or maybe I didn't want to believe—that there could be that much need for this information within my congregation. By the end of the next week, again all the tearoff sheets were gone. Then it dawned on me that our church facility is used by many groups within the community and I felt the Lord nudge me to begin an outreach to these organizations as well.

I contacted the Domestic Violence Center of Howard County as well as STAR (Sexual Treatment, Advocacy, and Recovery) Center for victims of sexual trauma. I also contacted the Sheriff's Department. I discovered that each of the facilities had different needs, which I thought we as a congregation could meet. The Domestic Violence Center of Howard County identified a need for paper products, cleaning supplies, sanitary supplies for women, soap, shampoo, hair conditioner, and body lotion. The STAR Center expressed a need for clean clothing. Many times when sexually traumatized women are treated at a hospital, their clothes are taken as evidence by the police. Even when the clothes are not confiscated by the police, the women don't want to wear the clothes that they had on when they were attacked. The clothing evokes painful memories and makes them feel unclean. As a result, the women have no clothing to wear out of the hospital. The STAR Center specifically requested underwear, sneakers, and jogging suits. I took these requests back to our church and several of the ladies' groups have taken this up as their mission. They bring these supplies to my office every week and I make sure they get to the shelters. In fact, I have a basket in my office where church members drop samples of soaps, shampoos, conditioners, lotions, and other toiletries that they pick up at hotels. I then pass these on to one of the shelters.

I called the Sheriff's Office and found out that they had a program to collect unused mobile phones. They take responsibility for getting batteries for the telephones and getting the phones charged. Even though the phone is not connected to a service provider as long as it is charged a call to 911 is always possible. The Sheriff's Office then distributes these phones to women and seniors who might need to make an emergency telephone call. Again my congregation has assumed this as another ministry project and on a regular basis I deliver unused cell phones to the Sheriff's Office.

In the past year I have been involved in coordinating the parish nurse/health ministry efforts in Howard County. As part of this role, I have made sure that each of the nurses from participating congregations receive the posters and information cards related to domestic violence, and many of them are also participating in the collection of used cell phones. During one of our network meetings, I arranged for a representative from the Domestic Violence Center to speak to the nurses and we watched the video *Broken Vows*, which looks at the problem of domestic violence from the perspective of different faith traditions.[4]

Terrill Stumpf's journey has taken him through many twists and turns, including serving as a parish nurse at Old First Presbyterian Church in San Francisco; at present he is the director of health ministry at Fourth Presbyterian Church in Chicago. Terry serves on the leadership teams of the Presbyterian Parish Nurse Task Force as well as the Presbyterians Against Domestic Violence Network; the Presbyterian Health, Education and Welfare Association; and Presbyterian Church (USA). Each of these positions extends the focus of his nursing journey beyond the church. For instance, at Old First Presbyterian he worked at a senior activity center. In his leadership roles in the Presbyterian Church, God has called Terry to serve and educate other parish nurses and to reach out to women who are trapped in abusive situations. Let's listen as Terry tells a story about his journey into domestic violence prevention.

I developed a worship service focusing not only on the effects of domestic violence, but also on God's response to the pain, suffering, brokenness, and frequently deaths that result from domestic violence. I emphasized that God's intention for the world is that we do no wrong or commit no acts of violence against one another. The worship service is intended to encourage participants to lift up the silent voices of those who live daily in fear or actual violence to themselves and their children. Because of the intense emotional tone of the worship service, some in attendance may experience strong psychological responses and feel the need to talk to someone during or following the service. I made sure that this support service was provided. Participants were encouraged to light a candle for someone that they hold in their hearts who is or has been touched by domestic violence. The worship service is structured to include a combination of relevant scripture readings, musical selections, prayers for healing, a Unison Prayer, a recitation of the Lord's Prayer, and, finally, dismissal. The visual background for the service was created using a display of T-shirts and a memory quilt obtained from the Clothesline Project in Chicago. This display bears witness to the violence against women. The quilt includes the names of women who have died because of domestic violence. The T-shirts hung around the room include white T-shirts for women who have died of violence; yellow or beige for women who have been battered or assaulted; red, pink, or orange for women who have been raped or sexually assaulted; blue or green for women who are survivors of incest or childhood sexual abuse; and purple or lavender for women attacked because of their sexual orientation. In addition to the visual display, playing softly in the background is the "Sounds of Silence," also created by the Clothesline Project. These sounds include a gong that is struck every ten seconds to acknowledge the battering of a woman that occurs every ten seconds in the United States; a whistle is blown at one-minute intervals to mark the rape of a woman every one minute in the United States; and a bell tolls every fifteen minutes to acknowledge the death of four women who are killed daily by men who supposedly loved them.

One morning I offered this worship as the morning prayer service at Fourth Presbyterian Church, where I am the director of health ministries. The invitation to worship is extended to the community at large as well as the staff and congregation of the church. Among the participants was a woman who is a member of the church. I could see that the service had a tremendous emotional impact on her, although she did not leave the service or seek individual counseling. Later in the day she came to my office and shared that the service had not only opened up wounds that she thought were healed, but had also brought necessary healing to these buried wounds. Throughout the service she was flooded with vivid memories of her mother's abuse at the hands of her father and then, later in life, her own abuse at the hands of her first husband. We talked and prayed together and she expressed a peace that she had not felt in a very long time. I am thankful that the Lord has taken me on a journey that leads to healing, reconciliation, and wholeness—both within the church congregation and beyond.

Journey of Hope to the "Greater Fifth Ward"

Dr. Karen Hahn, RN, APN, executive director of the Center for Faith and Health Initiatives in Seattle, Washington, wrote the following tribute to honor Shirley Branch, one of the parish nurses within the network that she oversees. Shirley has a vision for community, and despite a physical disability she mobilizes, energizes, and helps to move a damaged community to wholeness.

She can't walk too well, but she can fly. She flies with the wings of angels, her health ministry team. Her team members proudly call themselves "Shirley's Angels." I call her "Systa." She and her mother, Mama Moore, adopted me at a family reunion. I can't imagine doing faith community nursing without my Systa and my Mama. We have had ten years of learning, growing, and serving together. What makes my Systa so special? Two words tell why—her love and listening. This short story tells how these virtues transformed faith community nursing in Houston.

I first met Shirley at the faith community health coalition's first visioning meeting. Shirley's neighborhood was recovering from the devastating flooding of Tropical Storm Alison. Shirley was also recovering.

Tropical Storm Alison had crippled the Fifth Ward, a historic African American neighborhood. Damaged homes and businesses molded and crumbled. Pastors and members struggled to put their lives back together.

Alison had also disabled Shirley. Flooding had trapped her in her home and infected her leg. Depression dragged Shirley down after she could no longer work as a charge nurse on a medical floor. Cellulitis had damaged her leg so much that walking was difficult for her, even with a cane. However, Shirley took charge of her life and dragged her bum leg up a flight of stairs to get to that visioning meeting. She had been serving her own faith community, Fifth Ward Missionary Baptist Church, as a faith community nurse for over ten years. She was not going to miss this opportunity to work with other churches in her neighborhood.

Shirley Branch listened to the lively discussion about a health coalition of churches in the Fifth Ward for two hours. She quietly summed up everything with a few words: "Fifth Ward Congregational Health Coalition—Brings healing of the body and spirit to the community."

She knew her neighborhood needed hope. She suggested the logo of the dove carrying the branch, the image of hope to Noah after the flood. That logo carried the message of the coalition: hope and healing. The olive branch of hope helped rebuild the Fifth Ward.

Shirley was that branch. That early small coalition of two pastors in one neighborhood branched out to fifteen churches and now serves several neighborhoods. Now we joke: What do a tropical storm, a flood, a branch, and a roof have in common? Shirley Branch. You see, the olive branch was not the only branch in this story.

During Alison, a branch had fallen through the roof of Mrs. Gloria Jack's home, a founding elder of the Greater Fifth Ward Congregational Health Coalition. Mrs. Jack had begged FEMA and city agencies to fix that roof. This seventy-eight-year-old came to every coalition meeting and at every coalition meeting for three-and-a-half years she asked for help. She said her home was rotting away from a roof that continued to leak.

What could the coalition do? The city and home restoration agencies had refused to fix her home because they said it was beyond repair and needed to be torn down. This widow was convinced that the coalition would and should do something because she kept asking.

Shirley listened. She pointed out that the seniors who came to the coalition's Back-to-School Health Fair stopped at the coalition table every year to ask for help with repairs. She asked the coalition to look into home repairs for seniors.

The coalition did not jump to respond to this challenge. No one had money to buy supplies. No one was a roofer. Who would pay for damages if someone got hurt or someone sued? The Fifth Ward was littered with blighted and abandoned homes. It had the highest percentage of seniors in the city. Where and how could they choose which homes to fix?

Most of the coalition volunteers were seniors themselves. They knew how important home restorations were to neighborhood safety. Many had construction skills. They knew who really needed the help. They decided to revitalize their community.

The coalition formed the Caring Communities Home Restoration Project to coordinate partners and volunteers. They agreed to advocate with the city to replace Mrs. Jack's home. They also agreed to restore one home to try out the process.

Shirley's Angels—her mother, the coalition volunteers, and her church volunteers—adopted Caring Communities' first client. Mrs. Perry was a ninety-three-year-old childless widow who lived alone. She had paid caregivers but no living family left in the state, and no visitors. Caring Communities' volunteers not only saved her home from demolition, but also reconnected her to the community.

Mrs. Perry had not been out of her home for four years because she needed a wheelchair ramp. Her home needed much more than a ramp; the home needed a new roof, rewiring, kitchen plumbing, doors, and a full paint job. Her caregivers were hauling water from the tub to the kitchen to wash dishes and cook food. Her electrical wiring was dangerous because of the leaking roof.

One month later, Mrs. Perry had a beautifully restored home, a hospital bed, and visitors twice a week. A coalition pastor visited her every Sunday and brought her communion once a month. Mama Moore visited her every week and brought her news and food. The coalition was energized. They wanted to help more of their seniors.

In the next three years, the Caring Communities Home Restoration Project worked with four of the pastors near Shirley's church, renovated sixteen homes, and built sixteen wheelchair ramps. Habitat for Humanity built sixteen homes. They had revitalized one section of the Fifth Ward.

However, the persistent widow continued to remind the coalition that her home was still rotting away and the ceilings were falling down. The coalition enlisted an elected official and a TV investigative reporter as advocates to get her home replaced. The widow made daily calls to the city and worked with the coalition until her home of thirty-eight years was successfully demolished and a new one built.

Shirley's listening to the widow and other seniors in the community resulted in homes being renovated and replaced, and ramps being built. Like the persistent widow in scripture, Shirley would not take "no" for an answer.

Shirley knew that nothing is impossible when people of faith work together. She listened to what the community needed and wanted to do. She knew that love truly transforms. She insisted that *Caring Communities* was just as important as *Home Restoration Project* and made sure they stayed together.

She has loved and served her faith community and neighborhood for over thirty years. When dozens of homeowners fled her neighborhood and church because of highway and tollway construction, and then the threat of a railroad takeover, she stayed. She lived that covenantal love of faith community/parish nursing. Shirley has stayed through many threats to her community—severe poverty, crime, neglect, abandonment, and storms. Alison was the first of many storms. Much of the Fifth Ward is in a flood zone. After Alison came Hurricanes Rita, Katrina, and Ike. She and Mama Moore turned these and other storms into opportunities to mobilize their neighborhood.

They started Revere Corps, an organization of about a hundred seniors who get the word out about disaster preparedness. Named for Paul Revere, Revere Corps is rooted in respect for elders. Its strength is reverence for seniors and their role in the community. Almost half of the Revere Corps seniors are also FEMA Citizens Emergency Response Trained (CERT). The Revere Corps meets quarterly for networking, disaster role-plays, and trainings. Some have done disaster drills in their churches.

All Revere Corps members help make sure that seniors and family members have disaster plans, with special attention to vulnerable elders. Both Shirley, age sixty, and Mama Moore, age eighty, are disabled. As vulnerable seniors and respected leaders themselves, they know they can and need to make a difference. They know they make things happen by their example.

Shirley turned what could have been a tragedy in her life into a blessing for all. The storm of her disability became the motivation to redirect her leadership skills from the hospital setting to her neighborhood. She used her skills in her own faith community to help forge other churches and organizations into a community committed to working together.

She and her mother, Mama Moore, agreed to become Volunteers in Service to America (VISTAs) to try out a government capacity-building model in congregational health ministry. They each served as VISTAs for the full three years and helped to recruit and inspire others to work as VISTAs for coalition churches and organizations. Their leadership and example over the years attracted other VISTAs and kept the coalition strong and growing.

The Greater Fifth Ward Congregational Health Coalition, which Shirley helped to found, has become the oldest and largest faith-based health coalition in the Houston area. The coalition is now an organization of thirty-five-plus churches, health care organizations, and agencies that actively work together to bring healing of the body and spirit to the community. The coalition's volunteers have been giving more than seven thousand hours in community service each year for almost ten years. They give free senior and caregiving support services, congregational nursing, health, nutrition support, leadership development, home restoration, ramp building, and disaster management services, which are valued at more than $500,000 every year!

The Greater Fifth Ward volunteers are now on a mission to help others make a difference in their communities. Caring Communities volunteers have restored 20 homes, built 137 wheelchair ramps, and replaced 2 roofs. The Caring Communities Home Restoration Project has spread to three cities.

Shirley's love for her community and her listening have transformed faith community health nursing in Houston. Faith community health nursing truly has extended to the larger community—across faith communities. Rooting community health nursing in the deep, shared faith of the Fifth Ward has shown how building on the strengths of challenged communities can mobilize and transform them. Faith moves mountains—and communities.

The stories of these nurses are a reminder of God's depth and breadth. His call to nurses is not limited to a particular church or congregation. He calls nurses to be yeast and light to a broken world—yeast to multiply and expand works of compassion, concern, and care, both within and beyond congregational walls—and light to illuminate the needs that are there to be met, the talents of people who can meet these needs, and the path to be taken. In the refrain of a hymn titled "Jerusalem, My Destiny," written by Rory Cooney, the sentiment of a journey led by God is aptly captured: "I have fixed my eyes on your hills. Jerusalem, my destiny! Though I cannot see the end for me, I cannot turn away. We have set our hearts for the way; this journey is our destiny. Let no one walk alone. The journey makes us one."[5]

Thus far we have focused on how God calls nurses and their response to His call as He leads them on a journey to faith community/parish nursing and beyond. In the next chapter we shift our attention to the preparation needed for these journeys. It is said that God does not necessarily call those who are prepared but that He prepares those He calls. Let's take a look at how God prepares parish nurses.

5. Preparation for the Journey

Most people embarking on a new journey seek advice from others who have taken a similar path. We want to know the opportunities and the pitfalls. We want guidance as to how we should proceed and a warning about any dangers along the way. Commencement exercises traditionally feature speakers who point graduates in the direction of fulfillment. Anna Quindlen, a Pulitzer Prize–winning columnist, wrote a commencement speech for the graduates of Villanova University. Although she never gave the speech, it was published as *A Short Guide to a Happy Life*[1] and earned a long-standing place on the *New York Times* best-seller list. The phenomenal success of this book gives a glimpse into our longing for mentors and guides. Quindlen reminds readers that life is limited, and that we need to make the most of it and devote ourselves to meaningful activities.

Another enormously successful book, *Tuesdays with Morrie*[2] provides readers with the insights of Morrie Schwartz, a sociology professor who was dying of ALS. Morrie's shared wisdom focused on death, fear, greed, society, forgiveness, and a meaningful life. Schwartz noted, "People see me as a bridge. I'm not as alive as I used to be, but I'm not dead yet. . . . I'm on the last great journey here—and people want me to tell them what to pack."

This quest for mentors and guides derives from a rich religious heritage. Ancient Hebrews believed that living a good and happy life in community with neighbors and God was something that could be learned. Proverbs, psalms, and stories were used to teach successive generations of Israel's children the secrets of a rewarding life.[3] Today many still look to scripture for wisdom, guidance, and truths that can aid us in making life both more meaningful and more manageable.

Nurses who embark on the journey into parish nursing have already taken the advice of Quindlen, Schwartz, and countless biblical writers who point us away from self to a focus on others. Who are the mentors for parish nurses? Who are the adventurers who share their wisdom to light the way for the parish nurse journey? How does God prepare the nurses who are called to parish nursing? These questions are answered by examining the roots of the parish nurse movement and by exploring how those roots have expanded and evolved since 1984 when Reverend Granger Westberg formalized the concept of parish nursing. Reverend Westberg led the way, but he forged a path that has been further cleared by countless other nurse-leaders. This chapter looks at several of these leaders and the contributions they have each made to parish nurse preparation.

Reverend Granger Westberg

Let's go back to the earliest days of parish nursing and listen to the voice of Reverend Granger Westberg as he responds in an interview published in the 1989 issue of the *Journal of Christian Nursing*.[4] Reverend Westberg traced the beginnings of the parish nurse concept to an experience he had as the pastor of a church in Illinois in 1940.

One day at a Lutheran pastors' conference in Chicago, several other young ministers and I sat with the seventy-seven-year old chaplain of Augustana Lutheran Hospital. In the course of our conversation, this chaplain explained that he needed to be away from the hospital for a week. "Would one of you fellows like to take my place?" he asked. "I'd like to do that," I said. "I think it would be fun." That was the beginning of one of the greatest weeks of my life.

I was able to minister to patients effectively in a very short time. When people are lying horizontally in a hospital bed, they begin to think about the vertical dimension of life. They wonder about the meaning of life and start asking spiritual questions. But there's usually no one around to help them deal with those difficult questions, so they don't get very far in their thinking.

All during that life-changing week, I came in contact with people who needed help to think deeply and productively. I hope I helped them, as I injected biblical concepts into their thinking.

Just over three years later, as a result of contacts made that week, I became the chaplain at Augustana. That was 1944. I was thirty years old then, and people were just beginning to see the potential for changing lives through hospital ministry.

Over the years, ministering and teaching at Augustana and then at the University of Chicago, I began to see that a person's physical well-being was tied to his or her emotional and spiritual health. Again and again, as I talked to patients, I found that their illnesses seemed to originate in some personal struggle, often related to grief.

I felt that the key to preventive medicine lay in picking up people's early cries for help. Someone needed to be on the scene in the church to deal with people before they became seriously ill.

From these understandings, Reverend Westberg developed a wholistic health center to provide health care in a poor community.

We opened up a free clinic in a church, signed up two volunteer doctors and one volunteer nurse, and used seminary students to do counseling. Subsequently, we set up clinics in middle- and upper-income communities where people paid standard fees for the services. A nurse, a doctor, and a pastor would treat these people's complaints wholistically, recognizing that their problems stemmed from and affected not only the body, but also the mind and spirit.

But these clinics were expensive to start and operate. We had to pay the salaries of three or four professionals and the cost of renovating a building. And we had to subsidize operations because we couldn't charge a high-enough fee to cover the expense of treatment by three people instead of just one. However, a dozen of these clinics are still in operation across the country.

I realized that the nurse was the key member of the professional team in these clinics. So far all of them have been women. She had the sensitivity—the peripheral vision, I call it—to see beyond the patient's problems and verbal statements. She could hear things that were left unsaid. And she was the best listener.

For example, when we would conduct initial interviews with patients, it was the nurse who really heard what was said. Then afterward she would give feedback to the doctor and the pastor. "Do you remember when Mrs. Olson was starting to tell you something, and you butted in and gave a little sermonette, Doctor or Pastor? She had something important to say, I think, and you stopped her."

Nurses seem to have one foot in the sciences and one in the humanities, one foot in the spiritual world and one in the physical world. The nurses I've had the privilege to work with have been very perceptive; they have great insight into the human condition.

So many nurses I work with have a deep spiritual desire to help people. They don't view the hospital as a warehouse for sick bodies. They see people as sacred in God's eyes. Consequently, they look at the whole person, not just the ailment.

When many doctors enter a patient's room, too often they view the patient with a sort of tunnel vision. They see the physical problem and nothing else. If the patient has something wrong with his or her arm, doctors will go right to the arm, take care of it, and leave. Maybe they spend only a few minutes with that person. In many cases they say almost nothing to the patient beyond asking about physical symptoms.

But nurses entering the same room will see and hear a great deal more than some doctors. Nurses may comment on pictures or get-well cards, or talk with family members who've come to visit—all at the same time that they are caring for the patient's physical needs.

One day, while lamenting the expense of running a wholistic health center, a friend said, "You keep saying such wonderful things about nurses. Instead of opening a clinic, what if we just put a nurse on the church staff? Would that work?"

We tried it, and it worked. Then I approached the president of Lutheran Hospital in Park Ridge, Illinois, an old friend of mine. We discussed the concept of the parish nurse as a practitioner in preventive health care. He was as excited about it as I was. So we decided to test out the idea in six Chicago-area churches—four Protestant and two Catholic.

The six churches each chose a nurse. We gave them a list of applicants, and the congregations also had women who were interested in the positions. Lutheran General agreed to sponsor the program by paying 75 percent of the half-time salary for each nurse the first year. The second year the hospital paid 50 percent and 25 percent the third year. Thus, each year Lutheran General paid less and the churches paid an increasing percentage of their nurse's salary. By the fourth year, each church was paying the nurse's full salary.

Each year, as the hospital reduced its contribution to the original six nurses, we added two more churches to the program with the extra money. Now we have over twelve.

Thus began the first parish nurse programs. But what about parish nurse preparation? Was it enough to be a registered nurse or did Reverend Westberg find that additional preparation was required? Again, let's listen to his words.

We set up a low-key continuing education program at Lutheran General. Once a week the nurses met for half a day with me, the chaplains, a nurse from the hospital teaching program, and a doctor in family medicine. These people provided support and guidance for the nurses.

When we got together, the nurses shared stories about their ministry. Sometimes they role-played things that happened during the week. They exchanged ideas about ways to handle problems, and they had fellowship together and with the hospital chaplains.

When asked about the future of parish nursing, Reverend Westberg expressed a clear vision for this evolving nursing specialty. Let's listen to his wish list.

I'd like to have a thousand churches with parish nurse programs. We now have a Parish Nurse Resource Center at Lutheran General Hospital. I'd like to have a full-time director to run that. And, I'd like to see a special program for training parish nurses—either a six-week session at Lutheran General, or a staff member who would travel and train nurses on site.

Then I'd like to organize a parish nurse association to provide a newsletter and to set up local support groups for parish nurses. If I only had $35,000!

Reverend Granger Westberg had a clear vision. He started the journey toward establishing parish nurses in individual churches and parish nursing as a new specialty—one that truly focuses on whole-person health—physical, emotional, and spiritual. His vision and his wish list have all become realities. He took his vision and spoke across the country—to nursing groups, to nursing faculty teaching in Christian-based colleges and universities, and to hospital personnel. His mission was clear—to share the vision and to empower others to continue the journey he had begun.

Ann Solari-Twadell and the International Parish Nurse Resource Center

Unbeknownst to Reverend Westberg, God was orchestrating responses to Westberg's wish list across the entire country. Right in Westberg's backyard, Lutheran General Hospital hired Ann Solari-Twadell, former director of International Parish Nurse Resource Center, to work on a pilot project called Congregational Health Partnership. As Ann moved with uncertainty into her new role, she held onto the certainty that God had something important in mind for her. She was aware of this new concept of parish nursing. She knew that Reverend Westberg was sharing his vision nationwide and inspiring individuals to develop their own parish nursing programs. Ann was also aware that the original six parish nurses were being inundated with requests about "how to do it." The problem was that these requests were directed to nurses who were still in a pilot program themselves and were just beginning to discern the day-to-day operations of being parish nurses!

Ann recognized the need for resources and support for this growing movement. She went to her supervisor and proposed that Lutheran General establish a Parish Nurse Resource Center, which was endorsed in 1986. The center was formed out of the Office of Church Relations, Lutheran General Health Care System, in Park

Ridge, Illinois. An advisory board was formed, with local and national nursing and clergy representation. It was this group that recommended that a membership group be formed separate and independent from the Resource Center. This suggestion led to the formation in September 1988 of the Health Ministries Association, a membership group made up largely of parish nurses but open to all types of health ministers.

In September 1987, the Parish Nurse Resource Center offered the first continuing education program on parish nursing. This initial offering evolved into the annual Westberg Symposium on Parish Nursing. This symposium features preconference workshops on topics of current interest; a nurse is the keynote speaker and a major clergy presenter also offers thoughts on parish nursing. Abstracts for presentations and posters are solicited nationally as well as internationally. The conference includes worship and opportunities for networking, and produces a published book of proceedings that is distributed to all the participants. What began as a small local event, drawing 74 participants in 1987, has grown to an international event with about 1,000 participants from across the United States, Australia, Korea, Canada, England, and Ireland.[5]

In 1989 the Resource Center initiated a two-and-a-half-day continuing education program called Orientation to Parish Nursing. This program provided nurses with basic information regarding parish nursing, how to get started, and a discussion of legal concerns and accountability. Included within the orientation was a half-day of mentoring with one of the Lutheran General–sponsored parish nurses. This orientation program continued until 1996 when the Resource Center made a decision that initiation into parish nursing was best accomplished through Basic Preparation, a lengthier and more in-depth program. The Basic Preparation course was developed from the input of nurses representing educational institutions across the United States as well as from regional parish nurse networks.

In 1995, Lutheran General Health Care System was purchased by Advocate Health Care System and the Parish Nurse Resource Center was renamed the International Parish Nurse Resource Center to

---

Box 5.1   Core Curriculum Content for Basic Parish Nurse Preparation.
© 2010 Deaconess Parish Nurse Ministries, LLC.

	Hours
Unit 1: Spirituality	
1. History and Philosophy of Parish Nursing	2
2. Prayer	2
3. Self-Care	2
4. Healing and Wholeness	4
Unit 2: Professionalism	
1. Ethical Issues	2
2. Documenting Practice	2
3. Legal Aspects	2
4. Beginning Your Ministry	2
5. Communication and Collaboration	2
Unit 3: Wholistic Health	
1. Health Promotion	4
2. Transforming Life Issues: Family Violence	2
3. Transforming Life Issues: Suffering, Grief, and Loss	2
Unit 4: Community	
1. Assessment	2
2. Accessing Resources	2
3. Advocacy	2
4. Care Coordination	2
Total	36

---

reflect the expanding focus and influence of the center's work. The center has continued its efforts to standardize parish nurse preparation, to study organizational models and functions, and to provide resources for the development of quality parish nurse programs through research, education, publishing, and consulting. Currently, the International Parish Nurse Resource Center endorses two standardized courses for parish nurses: the Basic Parish Nurse Preparation

Course and the Parish Nurse Coordinator Course. Today there are approximately 140 providers across the country that have met the criteria established by the International Parish Nurse Resource Center to offer the curricula endorsed by the International Parish Nurse Resource Center. The content areas for each of these courses are detailed in Boxes 5.1 through 5.4.

Ann Solari-Twadell continues to contribute to the specialty of faith community/parish nursing. Since those early days of parish nursing, when she played such a significant role, she has earned a PhD and has focused her research and writing on spirituality, parish nursing, and spiritual care.

Box 5.2 Advanced Parish Nurse Coordinator Curriculum Table of Contents.
© 2010 Deaconess Parish Nurse Ministries, LLC.

Content Module	Hours
Unit I: Spirituality	
1. Self-Care for the Parish Nurse Coordinator	1½
2. Working with Diverse Faith Traditions	1½
Unit II: Professionalism	
3. Role of the Parish Nurse Coordinator	2
4. Documentation	1½
5. Human Resource Management	2
6. Professional Development of the Parish Nurse Coordinator	1½
7. Utilizing Research to Promote Best Practices	1½
Unit III: Wholistic Health	
8. Emerging Issues and Trends Impacting Parish Nursing	2
9. New Program Development	1½
Unit IV: Community	
10. Working with Faith Communities	1½
11. Funding and Grant Writing	1½
12. Growing and Sustaining Parish Nurse Programs	1½
13. Marketing and Promoting the Parish Nurse Program	1
Total Hours	20½

Box 5.3 Supplemental Modules 2005. © 2010 Deaconess Parish Nurse Ministries, LLC.

Module	Hours
1. Wholistic Health of Children	2
2. Wholistic Health of Adolescents and Young Adults	2
3. Wholistic Health of Middle Adults	2
4. Wholistic Health of Older Adults	2
5. Providing Spiritual Support	4–6
6. Sustaining and Nurturing the Parish Nurse Ministry	1½
7. Promoting Mental Wellness	3
8. Process of Theological Reflection in Parish Nursing	2
9. End-of-Life Transitions	2
10. Measuring Parish Nurse Ministry	2
11. Applying Leadership Skills in Parish Nurse Ministry	2
12. Conflict Resolution	2

Box 5.4 Supplemental Modules 2007

Module	Hours
1. Complementary Therapies: Overview	2
2. Complementary Therapies: Imagery	2
3. Complementary Therapies: Meditation	2
4. Tools and Techniques for Practice	2
5. Emergency Preparedness	2
6. Overview of Chronic Illness Management	2
7. Working with Rural Communities	2
8. The Social Justice Role of the Parish Nurse with Vulnerable Populations	2
9. Identifying Strengths of Congregations: Tapping into God's Power	2
10. Leadership Transitions in Congregations	2
11. Caring for Families	2

Rosemarie Matheus and Marquette's Parish Nurse Preparation Institute

While Ann was developing the Parish Nurse Resource Center, God was raising up other parish nurses and parish nurse preparation programs. Rosemarie Matheus was director of the Parish Nurse Preparation Institute at Marquette University College of Nursing until her retirement in 2003. Over the course of her career, she prepared over sixteen thousand parish nurses.

Rosemarie and a fellow faculty member, Dr. Richard Fehring, both attended a church meeting where the first parish nurses from Illinois were speaking. During this meeting, Rosemarie heard God call to her that she needed to develop a curriculum for parish nursing. Let's listen to Rosemarie share her wisdom about the specialty of parish nursing. Her observations come from her journey as an educator of parish nurses over ten years. She began to prepare a curriculum for parish nurses that was initially offered in 1990 at Concordia University in Mequon, Wisconsin. Nineteen nurses enrolled in Rosemarie's first class. This course was offered at Concordia for two years. Rosemarie then transferred the program to Marquette. In 1996, the Parish Nurse Preparation Institute was established and Rosemarie became the director.

People always assumed that I was a parish nurse—I felt that I was vicariously through all the nurses I trained over the years. When I began, there were so few nurses; I was working at Marquette and went to a presentation given by the original six parish nurses hired by Reverend Westberg. As I listened to these nurses speak, I just knew that they needed a structured program. So I worked with another faculty member, Dr. Richard Fehring, to develop a parish nurse curriculum. Richard moved away from parish nursing—his call was to natural family planning—but I stuck with Parish Nursing.

The first issue that we dealt with was "What should we teach?" We developed a questionnaire and distributed it to the fifty nurses who attended the Third Westberg Symposium and asked them what they needed. These nurses provided us with lots of information: They were already practicing in the role and had very definite ideas of what should be in the curriculum. Richard and I then embellished the curriculum from an educator's point of view.

I added components to the training, including campus living. I strongly encouraged the nurses to stay on campus and not to break up the educational experience by traveling home at the end of the day's instruction. Being together overnight really helped develop camaraderie. I made the training special and personalized it with little extras, like putting flowers in each of the dormitory rooms where the nurses stayed. I made individual greeting cards for each nurse with scripture verses written on the inside of the card. Many of the nurses would ask me how I chose the verses—they felt that their verses fit them perfectly. I quickly learned their names and called them by their names. I taught them how important it would be for them to learn the names of those they served within their churches. I developed a very personal relationship with the students: Even when I see some of them today, they tell me how meaningful the initial training was for them.

There were other things that I did to make the training personally meaningful. On Sunday afternoon, we would have a class and watch a video that stressed the importance to wellness of having fun and engaging in play—we went to Lake Michigan where we had a cookout and just enjoyed each other's company. On Tuesday night we would have a healing worship service—in the chapel dedicated to St. Joan of Arc. This chapel had great spiritual significance. Stone by stone it had been dismantled and sent from its original site in France. It is the only authentic medieval chapel in the Western hemisphere!

I explained that the healing had two purposes (healing services were not common and were considered a fringe activity at that time), yet healing is a tenet in most faith traditions. I would teach them, first, about the importance of healing and review the Book of James, where healing is clearly the role and responsibility of the church. I would show them how a healing worship service was done, and then I told them that the healing service was also for their own personal healing.

Recently, at a parish nurse support group, a parish nurse described her experience at one of those early worship services. I made each of them write a vow—not more than two or three sentences—about what they were learning and how they would use it in their own ministries. I held a commission service that lasted about an hour. Each of the parish nurses came with the vow she had written and I placed a ribbon on each of their necks—many of the nurses still have their ribbon. Also at the commission service, the nurses needed to bring a mission statement from their churches and they had to write how their parish nurse ministry would support that mission. They needed to present this information in front of their classmates. Most were unaware that their faith communities even had a mission statement and they were extremely uneasy about speaking in front of the group. However, I encouraged them and reminded them that speaking to the congregation would probably be part of their jobs as parish nurses. I made sure that the commissioning ceremony—in fact the entire curriculum—was spiritually rich.

I worked with Ann Solari-Twadell and Mary Ann McDermott to do the first curriculum review. We invited nurses from across the country and requested that they each write a module that Ann, Mary Ann, and I reviewed and edited to arrive at the first standardized curriculum. The original program was very intense and very different from the IPNRC curriculum that is taught today. The course ran seven to eight days from 7 a.m. until 4 p.m. The content was solid, but also diverse. We taught how parish nursing was a good fit for the Muslim mosque as well as the Jewish temple. We backed these assertions with readings from the Hebrew scriptures.

Most parish nurse ministries begin with a vision of establishing a healing community within a place of worship. The nurse is usually highly motivated and filled with ideas and plans to ensure success. What happens in the initial stages and in the months ahead is often predictive of the long-term success of the ministry. My work over many years with parish nurses and my interviews with experienced parish nurses have revealed a number of behaviors and actions that predict success or failure.

A primary step in the successful creation of a healing ministry within a congregation is to educate the congregants and the clergy that this ministry is grounded in scripture. Healing in the church is commanded by Jesus: "Heal the sick" (Matthew 10:8, Revised English Bible) and "He sent them out to proclaim the kingdom of God and to heal the sick . . ." (Luke 9:2). The church's mission, as these passages clearly state, is to heal. This process is not accomplished without patience, time (one to two years), and the devoted efforts of the nurse, the clergy, and congregants who want their place of worship to be a place of healing. M.I., a parish nurse of nine years, called it continually persevering. When D.S., a parish nurse of twelve years, started a program, she went to every group within the church and described it as a healing ministry based on scripture. A decision to start a parish nursing program, made only by the nurse and the clergy, and at times in collaboration with an outside agency such as a hospital, is *not* the optimal way to begin. First the congregation has neither ownership nor input in this ministry, which should reflect the mission of their church. Second, the onus of the ministry should not focus on one person—the nurse. This ministry must grow in the knowledge and practice that everyone in the congregation is a healer and in some way must be part of the healing ministry of the church.

To depend on the financial support of an outside health agency is very tempting and has been the deciding factor for many congregations. Experience has shown that in 80 percent of such start-up conditions, the health care agency will withdraw or alter its financial support due to budgetary constraints or a change in administration. To be a viable program for a health care agency, the program—in this case a ministry outside its walls—must show financial benefit, or in a few cases good public relations for the agency. This has been done in some parts of the country, but it is a time-consuming research task, not readily pursued by many parish nurses. Support of a parish nurse/healing ministry in a congregation by a health care agency is often erroneously misinterpreted as a clinic in the church, thereby losing its identity as a ministry directed by Jesus. Hospitals have admitted that their primary interest in supporting "clinics" in churches is to increase referrals to their facilities. Parish nurses may or may not be employees of the agency, and this can cause a conflict in establishing their interest. One hospital, for example, placed nurses in churches and set as their primary task to make follow-up calls to patients discharged from the hospital who lived within the churches' zip code, even when the person was not a member of the congregation.

Most long-term, successful parish nurse ministry programs derive financial support from the church's budget, which is often augmented by outside grants and personal donations. All the programs of a church are grounded in its mission—education, preaching, outreach. In order to be in alignment with the command to heal, the healing ministry of the church should be financed in the same manner as its teaching and preaching.

Nurses who see the position of parish nurse as a new, often easy job are diminishing the role. L.K., a parish nurse for ten years, pointed out that there are a lot of other (nursing positions) that would be a lot easier. Successful parish nurses are those who are responding to a calling from God to the healing ministry of the church. The call comes in different ways and at different times. For some, it was hard to hear for years because the din and busyness of their life drowned it out. For others, it wasn't heard until they found themselves pursuing the role and even then often denied that they were qualified. God doesn't call the qualified; God calls and then equips those called with the needed qualities. Were Matthew, a tax collector, or Peter, a fisherman, equipped to spread the message of Jesus when they were first called?

Parish nurses are required to work independently and use advanced nursing knowledge and strategies in complex situations. A church administrator attributed the success of the congregation's parish nurse to the fact that she had excellent problem-solving skills and extensive practical knowledge. One nurse considering a parish nurse position was told by the Department of Rehabilitation that nursing in a church would be an easy, nondemanding job. Believing this, she did not succeed in the role.

Because parish nursing is a specialized role within the profession, it is necessary for the nurse to complete a specialized parish nursing educational program. Similarly, nurses working in emergency departments and intensive care units are taught specialized skills beyond their basic nursing education. Parish nurse preparation programs vary with the agency that offers them, ranging from an inadequate, short orientation to a prolonged period of instruction, including the application of nursing as it pertains to the wholistic care of people. The spirit, mind, and body affect response to disease, self-care practices, and one's self-concept of valuing health.

While the clergyperson is ultimately responsible for all the ministries in the church, the clergyperson *cannot* be the parish nurse's supervisor. The clergyperson is knowledgeable about neither health care nor nursing concepts, and thus can neither judge nor decide on the appropriateness of the work of the parish nurse.

Congregations need to consider a number of factors before choosing a parish nurse, since the success of the parish nurse is a major predictor of the success of the ministry as a whole. Among the issues to take into account are these:

1. The nurse should be aware of and have a demonstrated belief in the paramount role of the spirit of each individual in preventing and healing illness. The candidate must be grounded in her own relationship with God. L.K., a parish nurse of ten years, told me that she chose the position because she had a desire to be a conduit between the parish members and God. The aspiring candidate needs to be aware of the difference between healing and curing. A person can be healed without being cured.

2. The nurse should be professionally in touch with the health needs of the community as identified in the goals of local, state, and national public health agencies, and work with them in their strategies. She needs to be aware of the latest advances in health care and needs to establish a collegial relationship with other health care providers in her area, and join any local parish nurse support and networking groups.

3. Successful parish nurses have come from a variety of nursing positions and experiences. A main determinant of success is the nurse's history and commitment to ongoing education. Too often, churches have selected a nurse who is a member of the congregation, without much thought and without being aware of the complex health care issues that its members are dealing with.

4. A major question I have been asked is this: Should the parish nurse be a member of her own congregation? In the majority of cases, my answer is no. It is not necessary for her to even belong to the same denomination. The focus of the parish nurse's work is the spiritual

life of the congregants, that is, their relationship with their God. It is not to teach, explain, or defend any theology. As a member of the congregation, the parish nurse comes with some "baggage," especially if she has been a congregation member for a number of years. She has probably formed friendships with other parishioners, which can hinder those parishioners from viewing the parish nurse as an objective or authentic health care provider. Every church has divisions, and without intent the parish nurse may be seen as part of a division that some parishioners view as "other." I've heard statements such as, "She was a favorite of the pastor" or "She always tries to change things." In one congregation with a large number of physicians and health care professionals, the parish nurse, an elderly, lifelong member, was described to me by the pastor as a nurse who knew little about current health care and as a result the ministry failed.

If the parish nurse ministry does not succeed in the congregation, it may create an awkward situation for both the nurse and the church. If it is due to her ineffective practice and she is asked to leave, must she also leave the church? Scripture alerts us to the possible consequences of practicing in one's own church: A prophet never lacks honor except in his hometown (Matthew 13:57).

I have placed nurses in churches other than their own church. These nurses have easily adapted to the new environment and been quickly accepted by the congregation. A Spanish-speaking Catholic nun was the parish nurse in a Baptist congregation with primarily Puerto Rican members. After several months she was called to the altar and awarded a certificate of appreciation for all the help and loving care she had given its members.

When several congregations mutually agree to have one parish nurse serve three or more congregations, this seemingly cooperative plan has not been successful. Health agencies frequently use this plan to demonstrate an agency's attempt at community service. Instead of practicing a health ministry guided by the church's mission, the parish nurse again becomes an employee of a health agency that provides superficial "band-aid" services during occasional drop-in visits. For a parish nurse practice to be successful, the nurse must be visible to the members, have a deep knowledge of their health needs, and form trusting relationships with them. This cannot be done when her "caseload" is potentially hundreds of members spread over several congregations. Serving two small to moderate-sized congregations is the limit to ensure success within the framework of parish nursing. R.H. believes that the success of her twelve years as a parish nurse is due to being seen and respected as a woman of faith and an active participant in the life of the church. On one occasion I strongly tried to warn five congregations about this potential problem. They ignored my advice and within one year, three of the congregations had dropped the program.

5. If the new parish nurse comes to her position with a mind frame of being all things to all people, and then attempts to perform and direct the entire healing ministry of a church, she will not succeed. Parish nursing is not a Lone Ranger position. The ministry must involve a large percentage of the members in the activities of the ministry, both in planning and carrying them out. Admittedly, this is difficult to achieve, and cannot be done overnight. Members will be quick to say, "I know nothing about health care." They need to be reminded that they are all consumers of health care. Most are also not aware of the distinction between healing and curing, and of the commandment to the church to be a place of healing. Educating members on these issues is essential for the success of the ministry. Visitation ministry, teaching wholistic health classes, creating a library of resources for members to learn about their disease, and self-care practice are just a few ways members can use their gifts to enrich the healing ministry.

6. For a strong beginning of the parish nurse program and the healing ministry, and as a demonstration of congregational support, a brief commissioning service has been successful. At this service, congregation members are visually introduced to this new person, hear the clergy support her ministry, and oftentimes she becomes a member of the ministerial team. This occurs after the governing board—and, in some cases, a vote by the members—has approved the ministry. A parish nurse should not begin to practice until this approval is given. In one case an overzealous nurse created a written brochure describing herself as the parish nurse before the board was aware of her plans, and even the clergyman had not yet given his support. When the clergyman became aware of the brochure, he announced to the congregation that "We do not have a parish nurse," and that church probably never will.

The reasons for the success or failure of parish nursing programs and health ministries are many and varied. These reasons became apparent to me during my years of teaching, mentoring, observing, and listening to parish nurses, clergy, and congregations of all faiths. Parish nurses of all ages are successful in all denominations and in congregations of all sizes. Success or failure is determined by the following factors:

- The interaction between the politics of a congregation and its approval.
- The support or lack of support by the clergy.
- The abilities, characteristics, and sensitivity of the parish nurse.
- Most importantly, basing the ministry on scripture's command that we are to teach and preach *and* heal.

Ruth E. Williams, Viterbo University

The following story comes from Ruth E. Williams, RN, MEPD, MSN, FCN/PN, from Viterbo University in Wisconsin. Ruth has been an active parish nurse for eighteen years, having first been trained by Rosemarie Matheus. Ruth went on to develop her own parish nurse training program at Viterbo.

The request for my story has prompted me to conduct a review of my practice at St. Mary's Church, where I go every Friday from 9 a.m. to noon. I never miss a Friday, except to teach parish nursing or to attend a parish nursing event. The Fridays I teach I schedule my office hours for Thursday morning. I try to visit other parishioners during the week. I have been practicing parish nursing for eighteen years. If there aren't any congregants to see during my office hours, I spend that time praying or doing office work. I am so blessed to have been able to teach parish nurses and to be a parish nurse ministering to the members of my church. I thank the Lord for all of this!

After attending Rosemarie Matheus's parish nursing class in June 1992 at Concordia University in Mequon, Wisconsin, I came home to St. Mary's of the Assumption Church in Richland Center, Wisconsin, and started my parish nurse ministry practice. At that time I was a faculty member at Viterbo University's Nursing Department in La Crosse, Wisconsin. In 1993,

I was asked by the Returning Registered Nurse Program coordinator to write a course on spirituality for nurses. This seemed very appropriate at the time. However, in writing about spirituality for nurses, I discovered that I had started to write the first course on parish nursing at Viterbo University, which was included in the Viterbo catalog as Nursing 300. This started parish nursing at Viterbo. This course consisted of five units on the following concepts:

1. the parish nurse's role in spirituality and healing;

2. wholeness, wellness, illness;

3. spiritual dimensions;

4. cultural dimensions; and

5. interpersonal and intrapersonal dimensions of parish nursing.

The first class I taught from this new curriculum was at St. Joseph's Hospital in Hillsboro, Wisconsin, with then Bishop Burke officiating at the very first dedication for parish nurses in the St. Francis Chapel in the hospital. I taught this course to many RNs between 1993 and 2000. In 2000, I attended the International Parish Nurse Resource Center (IPNRC) Faculty Preparation course, held at Divine Word Seminary in Techny, Illinois. There we received the more standardized modules for educating parish nurses internationally. This new course was taught in La Crosse, Hudson, Rice Lake, Janesville, Wausau, New Richmond, Reedsburg, Green Bay, Prairie du Chien, Eau Claire, Beloit, Rothschild, Richland Center, and Sparta (all in Wisconsin).

Since 2000, I have attended every yearly faculty retreat held at the IPNRC to keep updating my knowledge. I have also worked on the Research Committee. I taught the Parish Nurse Coordinator course at Baraboo and La Crosse. During that time I wrote and organized many retreats and updates for parish nurses, which are held at the Franciscan Spirituality Center in La Crosse, Wisconsin.

In 2002, I created a website, www.parishnurseheartland.com, which garners an average of 36,000-plus visits every year, reading about Viterbo University and parish nursing. The visitors to the site are from many countries, including the United Kingdom, Ireland, Canada, Egypt, Morocco, India, China, Japan, Russia, Germany, France, Brazil, Sweden, Norway, the Seychelles Islands, and even Christmas Island!

I wrote a book, called *A Collection of Parish Nurse Newsletters*, which was published in 2007 by the Dorrance Publishing Company in Philadelphia. Viterbo University has made history, broken new ground, and fostered new ideas for nursing, and parish nursing, in particular. Through the years since I started as a parish nurse-educator, our standards of practice have been incorporated into the American Nurses Association (ANA) *Scope and Standards of Practice.*

In my years at Viterbo, I believe we have educated over fifteen hundred parish nurses. These years have been very fruitful and rewarding for me. It is especially rewarding for me to see parish nurses I have taught, who are active in parishes, clinics, hospitals, nursing homes, and Catholic Residential Services (CRS) in the diocese of La Crosse and other states within the United States.

Reverend Dr. Deborah L. Patterson, Executive Director of Deaconess Parish Nurse Ministries, LLC, and the International Parish Nurse Resource Center

On January 1, 2002, Reverend Dr. Deborah L. Patterson became the executive director of International Parish Nurse Resource Center. She is also an ordained United Church of Christ minister. At the same time Deborah assumed leadership of IPNRC, the ownership of the IPNRC was transferred from Advocate Health Care, related to the Evangelical Lutheran Church in America and the United Church of Christ, to the Deaconess Parish Nurse Ministries, an entity of the Deaconess Foundation in St. Louis. This transfer included the annual Westberg Symposium, which is held in downtown St. Louis.[6]

Deborah has provided leadership for the IPNRC since 2002. Under her leadership the IPNRC has expanded its reach beyond the borders of the United States. In addition to being a regular contributor to *Parish Nurse Perspectives*—the online quarterly publication that is the only international periodical for parish nurses, Reverend

Dr. Patterson has written several books, including *Health Ministries* (2008), *Healing Words for Healing People* (2005), and *The Essential Parish Nurse* (2003).

The following text came from an interview with Deborah that appeared on the website HopeandHealing.org (HH), and provides a glimpse into her views and vision for faith community/parish nursing.

When I was a pastor serving a local congregation, I realized that most of my work was health-related. There were five women in our parish who were in a head-on collision on the highway and all ended up in intensive care at different hospitals in the area. I had all kinds of questions as I ran between the different ICUs. I wished that there had been someone in the church who could help me figure out what it meant if someone had a head injury. Or how to borrow durable medical equipment. Or how to help a family figure out if the physical therapy services in their area accepted their insurance. We needed more information to help us support the families as a congregation.

I had heard about parish nursing at that time and thought that would be a huge help to me in my ministry. There was also someone who was getting medicine from her doctor, what the patient called "nerve pills," to keep her sedated. I suggested that she get a second opinion and, when she got a second opinion, it turned out she had breast cancer. She was being sedated for symptoms of the disease. Another person had a daughter who was living in the basement of her home with obsessive-compulsive disorder (OCD). She kept washing her hands and could not leave the basement. So I helped that family get access to mental health resources, where the daughter got effective treatment. She was able to get out of the basement and get a job. I thought, "We are called to preach, teach, and heal, but this healing stuff is taking all my time in a way that I am not equipped to do?"

HH: Can you describe the role of a parish nurse?

They are registered nurses who have a minimum of two to three years' experience—enough that they can operate on their own. Most parish nurses bring ten to thirty years (or more) of experience to this position—

seasoned nurses are attracted to this profession. They are guided by the Faith Community Nursing Scope and Standards for Practice, published by the American Nurses Association. The parish nurse has seven roles:

1. Health educator

2. Health counselor

3. Advocate

4. Resource liaison

5. Developer of support groups

6. Coordinator of volunteers

7. Integrator of spirituality and health

Spirituality (#7) has to be woven through all the other roles.

HH: How do parish nurses integrate spirituality into their practice with a congregation?

Everything the parish nurse does must be an intervention desired by the client. Unless they have a huge parish, parish nurses serve both the people in their congregation and neighbors with related needs—a service of inreach and outreach. It is not "We only serve our own," but "We serve." We call our clients forth to articulate their own spirituality. When someone says, "Why me? Why would God do this to me?" it is about listening and asking, "Why are you asking that question?" A parish nurse finds out what is happening in the body and the spirit.

HH: Do you see a historical, biblical, or theological basis for the role of the parish nurse in a church?

Absolutely. As early as Acts 3, where you find ministries being divided up, some are called to go out and preach and some are called to go out and serve. This is clearly a ministry of service. Jill Westberg McNamara, following in the footsteps of her father, had this vision: Every home has a medicine cabinet, so every faith community should have a health cabinet with resources for those with a health need. We found that a parish nursing ministry is not a ministry of one person; it is a ministry of the congregation. That health cabinet is responsible for making this visible to the congregation. That health cabinet helps do the initial health survey of the congregation to find out the parishioners' health needs and interests. It also interprets parish nursing to the congregation—developing its form and function.

HH: How do parish nursing and congregational health ministry work together?

They have to work together; otherwise, it is just one nice little person making visits on the homebound. That may be one role of parish nursing, but to integrate spirituality and health, it means all of us work together; we are the body of Christ. If one suffers, we all suffer. This is all about inviting, empowering, and equipping others to participate. There is a Catholic parish in Cape Girardeau, Missouri, where the parish nurse has the luxury of having three hundred health professionals as members of that parish whom she can call on to help with health ministry. It is a large Catholic parish that is near a large medical center in Cape Girardeau. Basically, all the doctors and nurses belong to that congregation. She is able to help pull folks together to make all kinds of thing happen. In Texas, there is another parish nurse who serves a very large parish where there are social workers, teachers, and other gifted people to work in their growing health ministry.

People who have received the services of a parish nurse ministry are the people who want to volunteer. They want to serve in the way they were served. They are the best volunteers and the best financial supporters because they have seen and felt the work of this ministry—a ministry that is often invisible to many.

Last year I fell down and fractured my back. We were very lucky to have a parish nurse in my home congregation. She came to look at the medications prescribed by different doctors to look for any possible interactions; she identified some warning signs of drug interactions. She showed me how to get in and out of bed correctly and surveyed my home environment for any safety hazards that I was more susceptible to because of my injury. She brought over medical equipment from the church. This same care should be available to anybody in any congregation and any of their neighbors. Who is not a neighbor to a church some-where? Here it is available for anyone and there is no charge.

HH: How do you see the future of parish nursing and health ministry?

For the future, parish nursing must pursue evidence-based practice. A study of four hundred spouses and caregivers, conducted at New York University's Silverman Aging and Dementia Research Center, indicates that when the caregiver receives strong support, the person who is ill can generally stay at home for eighteen months longer, rather than being placed in a nursing home. To provide this support, often the parish nurse and the clergy will make a home visit together. The nurse can care for the person who is very ill and the pastor may go for a walk with the caregiver to provide support. Having that kind of data allows us to build this profession and show what a difference we make.

Dr. Norma Small and Dr. Ruth Stoll

Dr. Norma Small, former associate dean for graduate studies and director of gerontologic and adult health nursing, School of Nursing, Georgetown University, and Dr. Ruth Stoll, a former professor of psychiatric nursing at Messiah College in Grantham, Pennsylvania, represent two of the earliest forerunners in parish nurse preparation and each has a story to tell. Both Norma and Ruth heard Granger Westberg speak at Messiah College in 1988. They met and spoke with Granger Westberg while he was at Messiah College and Norma commented that the evolving role of the parish nurse called for an advanced practice nurse. Norma shares:

A year after my conversation with Reverend Westberg, I read an announce-ment that he had made in a Lutheran newsletter. Much to my surprise, he announced that Georgetown was beginning a parish nurse specialty in its master's program! I showed this announcement to the dean of the School of Nursing, who gave me approval to develop and submit to the faculty a curriculum plan for parish health nursing as a new specialty in the graduate program. The faculty approved parish health nursing as a new specialty in 1989 and the first student was admitted in 1990. The program consisted of thirty-six hours of master's-level courses. Twelve hours (three four-credit courses) were devoted to the specialty of parish nursing. These courses included the theory behind promoting health, the integration of spirituality into wholistic nursing practice, and a parish nurse practicum. Students were encouraged to take electives in theology, spiritual direction, and courses related to their specific faith tradition. Georgetown forged an agreement with Washington Theological Union to open courses to graduate students in parish health nursing.

One of the major obstacles that Norma faced was finding a suitable site where students could complete the practicum in parish nursing.

At that time the closest parish nursing program was in Harrisburg, Pennsylvania, approximately a three-hour drive from Georgetown University. So I developed a parish nursing program at Christ Lutheran Church, located on 16th Street in Washington, D.C. I served the congregation for three years as a parish nurse while I provided mentoring for my students in their new roles. Three parish nurses graduated from this program. Unfortunately, Georgetown closed the program in 1993 because of the cost and at that time there was a very limited market for master's-prepared parish nurses.

Norma is retired from Georgetown, but not from parish nursing. She continues to teach her own course for parish nurses and health ministers. The course is presented for thirty-five hours of continuing education credits in Johnstown, Pennsylvania. Every summer Norma also presents the course at Otterbein College in Columbus, Ohio. When the course is offered at Otterbein, it is offered for both continuing education credits as well as for undergraduate and graduate credits. She was awarded the 2003 HMA Wilkerson-Droege Award in recognition of her groundbreaking efforts with Health Ministries Association (HMA)—Norma was a charter member—as well as for her pioneering work on the initial *Scope and Standards of Parish Nursing Practice*, published in 1998.[6]

After Dr. Ruth Stoll heard Reverend Westberg speak at Messiah

College, she was also motivated to develop a course in parish nursing. Ruth describes her initial efforts in 1990 as a "stab in the dark"—there was so little concrete material to work with related to curriculum development.

Jan Towers, another doctorally prepared nurse faculty member at Messiah, and I began a year-long course that resulted in the awarding of a certificate in parish nurse practice. Through the end of 1991, thirteen students met with us once every two weeks. The content of the course focused on promotion and preventions of disease and spiritual interventions. Dr. Towers did not choose to continue with the course.

Jo Sensenig, a parish nurse in a nearby Mennonite church, had a master's degree in community health nursing and was very active in the Mennonite Health Ministry. Jo and I revised the initial course. We soon discovered that the course needed more time and structure. In 1992 we developed six continuing education courses based on what we believed were the key issues in parish nursing. We taught these courses in evening and Saturday format. Our first class of five nurses completed the courses and received a certificate of completion from Messiah College. This format continued through 1996.

In addition to the certificate course offered at Messiah College, we instituted an annual parish nurse conference. Conferences serve as another modality through which God prepares nurses who are called to parish nursing. In 1992, the conference began as a one-day meeting with a keynote speaker, workshops, and opportunities for networking. By 1996 the conference had evolved into a two-day meeting held each June. Jo and I collaborated with Holy Spirit Hospital and a task force of parish nurses and pastors to sponsor the event. The impact of the conference was greater than we ever anticipated. By 1996 we had at least six hundred names on our mailing list with over one hundred people in attendance at each conference. The opportunities for networking and sharing of information were tremendous. Nurses still tell me how valuable the conferences were!

Today Dr. Ruth Stoll is still actively involved in parish nurse education. The parish nurse basic course has been taught through a number of institutions in Pennsylvania—Lycoming College and Guthrie Health Care System, both in Williamsport; Hershey Medical System, in Hershey; and presently through Samaritan Counseling Center in Lancaster.

In addition to the Parish Nurse Basic Course and the International Parish Resource Center Curriculum, Ruth offers expanded content and hours of instruction to include more on spiritual foundation, theology of health and healing, spirituality and whole-person health, integration of faith and health, values and ethics in health ministry, spiritual wholeness, and spiritual care.

After completion of five units of Clinical Pastoral Education at Hershey Medical Center, Ruth began teaching the Parish Nurse Basic Course at Hershey Medical Center under the auspices of the Department of Pastoral Care and the Department of Nursing Education. This cooperative effort allowed for both a certificate of completion for the curriculum approved by the International Parish Nurse Resource Center and continuing education credits approved by the Pennsylvania State Nurses Association (ANA approved). In the last three years, Ruth has been facilitating and teaching the course offering in Lancaster, through the Samaritan Counseling Center. It is evident that the outreach to the course participants has become regional in scope. The participants come from all over the south-central region of Pennsylvania. At this time, more than seventy nurses and lay health ministers have been commissioned through our Parish Nurse Basic Course in this region. In addition, we have collaborated with Deb Best, Coordinator of Health Ministry in the Upper Susquehanna Lutheran Synod, Williamsport, in offering the course simultaneously in Lewisburg, Pennsylvania. This has nearly doubled the nurses who have become certified in this region of Pennsylvania. Opportunities and challenges are endless! God is faithful!

Dr. Eleanor Edman: A "Connector of People"— The Northwest Conference

We were encouraged by Wanda Alexander (see Chapter 4) to contact Dr. Eleanor Edman; Wanda described Eleanor as a "connector of people" who had been a tremendous resource to the parish nurse movement in Minnesota. Dr. Eleanor Edman retired as program chair and professor emeritus of the Bethel University Nursing Department in 1997 and has remained active in the faith community/parish nurse movement ever since her retirement. She minimizes her contributions to the specialty and points to others who, in her words, "have done so much more." Eleanor describes the role of the Northwest Conference Parish Nurse Commission.

I have done a lot since my retirement, but I am not in charge of anything. I am still on the Parish Nurse Commission, which is part of the Evangelical Covenant Lutheran Church of the NW Conference [includes Minnesota, parts of Wisconsin, Iowa, and South Dakota].

Eleanor continues with an overview of the role of the NWC:

The NWC Commission continues to act as coordinator, resource provider, consultant, and supporter to the nurses and congregations of the conference. Members are drawn from all geographic areas of the conference region to represent rural and urban churches as well as small and large congregations. Policies are in place to define membership, terms of office, officers, goals and activities, and mission statement. Commission activities and programs include the following:

• Meet regularly to plan activities, keep in touch with nurses, and continue to provide information and assistance to developing ministries.

• Make funds available to congregations for the start-up of a new ministry.

• Consult with congregations wishing to learn more about parish nurse ministry.

• Plan and conduct an annual fall retreat at Covenant Pines for nurses and other interested health care ministry volunteers. Programs have covered such topics as:
  Mental health issues related to teens and their families
  The ministry of healing and wholeness
  Dealing with abuse in the family
  Health care legislation
  Spirituality and the parish nurse

- Provide information and scholarships or support for nurses to attend national seminars and conferences, such as the Westberg Symposium, congregational health seminars at the Covenant Midwinter Conference, and parish nurse preparation programs.

- Be available to give reports, host an information booth, and provide updates on the ministry to the annual meeting or other gatherings of NW Conference churches.

Wanda Alexander stated that Eleanor possesses an uncanny ability to see strengths in others of which they are totally unaware, and once she identifies these gifts she is able to persuade those individuals to use them. In 2009 Eleanor wrote a wonderful article, titled "Out of the Clinic and into the Church,"[7] in which she recounts the history of the Northwest Parish Nurse Commission. In this article, true to her humble nature, Eleanor shines the light on the accomplishments of the individuals who have made this Parish Nurse Commission so successful. For instance:

Mary Gardeen and Carolynn Lundgren from First Covenant in Minneapolis work together and recently wrote about a unique day in their ministry: "It wasn't planned this way, but in a single day we visited the oldest and the youngest member of our congregation. The first visit came at the request of a family who said, "Please come. She is near the end. Our mother is in a health care facility and is failing rapidly." The nurses were able to help make this gentle, but agitated child of God more comfortable because of a conversation with the staff nurses about what they observed, then pray with the family as the staff continued to provide care."

The second visit was to a family with a newborn baby. They said, "One book was closing while the second book was just opening to the first page. In the first visit, we prayed for peaceful release for the dying mother and comfort for the family. During the second visit we admired the baby, congratulated the parents, and prayed for all that lay ahead. In the tradition of the biblical deaconess Phoebe, we ministered to both the physical and spiritual health needs of these families."

In another situation the parish nurse assisted the pastor in ministering to a family in a crisis situation. A church member, who was well known to the nurse, had experienced severe chest pains in the middle of the night. He lived alone, did not realize how serious his condition was, and drove himself to the Emergency Room of a nearby hospital. When he arrived, it was very clear that his condition was critical. His adult children and the pastor were called. The problem was that the family did not know what their father's wishes were regarding life-support measures. Shortly after admission, he became unconscious. The pastor called the parish nurse and asked if she had any information that would help in this difficult situation.

The nurse had recently held classes on Advanced Directives and had kept copies of these papers on file. She had a copy of this man's directive in her file, which she brought to the Emergency Room so that his wishes could be followed. He passed away later that day. The family and the pastor were so grateful for the way their father, and the pastor's parishioner, was cared for both by the hospital and the church staff.

An episode at a morning coffee hour illustrates how the role of the nurse was viewed at another church. A group of older women brought the parish nurse to the table of one of their friends and said, "Will you tell Esther to please see her doctor at the clinic tomorrow? She isn't feeling good, she is getting worse, and she won't listen to us." The nurse took their friend to her office, listened to her story, took her blood pressure, asked some questions, and gently urged her to see her doctor at the clinic as soon as possible. The nurse offered to go with her if she did not want to go alone. This is a typical occurrence when the parish nurse is known and respected.

Carol Story and Puget Sound Parish Nurse Ministries

Carol Story, the director of Puget Sound Parish Nurse Ministries, is another leader in parish nurse preparation. Let's listen to her story.

Actually my story begins with simply becoming a nurse. Little did I know that every step in my career would lead me to become a parish nurse-educator and program coordinator for a ministry! As I review my career—from my first job in the hospital working with all female patients, to being a supervisor in surgery, to office nursing, and even being an information and assistance worker for Senior Services—I can see how God has graciously led me though it all to be in this place at this time in my life. And I love it! I didn't become a Christian until I was thirty-two years old! He does work in mysterious ways.

My adventure in parish nursing began in 1992 when I attended a one-week intensive parish nursing class in Wisconsin. I came home excited and eager to begin a program in my church, but also with the thought of finding a means to begin an educational program for nurses who were interested in the concept. I continued to pray that God would give me direction and wisdom about where to go with the educational aspect that seemed to dominate my thoughts. I had not shared this with others because my reasoning was "Who am I?" and "Who would listen to me or take a class that I developed?" However, I received support and encouragement from my former dean, who had engaged another student and me in researching the concepts of parish nursing. Today she is still an encourager!

God truly pulled strings to get me into graduate school (my GRE scores were terribly inadequate—I'm a lousy test taker!), where I decided to go into program development and community health. Interestingly, I stumbled into a situation that made it possible for me to do my thesis work on spirituality and spiritual need (this was a secular university). I had the privilege of meeting and talking with an author of this book, Verna Carson, while at an NCF conference in the summer of 1992, when I took the parish nursing class. She also encouraged me to do the thesis work on spirituality. This is what really hooked me on the concept of parish nursing. I had a very strong sense that if nurses were going to work in churches, it was imperative that they (and I) understand the concept of spiritual care, spiritual need, and appropriately sharing their faith—even in their own congregations. Later, this same conviction led me to take a unit of clinical pastoral education. This was a decision that really changed my life and my walk with the Lord.

Soon after completing graduate school, I was invited to attend a meeting with nurses interested in parish nursing. Some of these nurses had taken an introductory course. When the leader, Dr. Ken Bakken, asked for a volunteer to coordinate some future meetings for this group, I agreed to do so—if at least four others would, too. I remember telling the Lord that I would be willing to do whatever he wanted to spread the word about parish nursing—anything except speak in front of groups! The five of us met on a regular basis and we spent most of the meetings in prayer. I met with potential speakers and one of them said, "Why don't you develop an educational course for parish nurses?" I looked at him with a blank stare and then shared how God had given me that very goal many months before. Then he said he would write the pastoral care section. He was sure that Dr. Bakken, who had published a book on wholeness and healing in the Christian tradition, would write the section on Theology of Healing and Health. Suddenly, our group had a purpose: to provide education and support for nurses interested in parish nursing!

We submitted the course to the Washington State Nurses Association and received approval for sixty-two continuing education units. We held our first class in September 1994. Later we were invited to affiliate with Pacific Lutheran University. This allowed us to offer participants the option of receiving college credits or continuing education units. About this time I read a publication from the Parish Nurse Resource Center that listed suggested content for parish nursing courses. I was delighted to discover that the research and groundwork that my friend and I had done in 1992 had paid off: We exceeded those recommendations with the content we were offering in our course. Today, we partner with the International Parish Nurse Resource Center in the IPNRC's continuing effort to standardize content and criteria for entry into practice. We have ten faculty, each an expert in the content that they teach, blending their knowledge with the concepts of parish nursing. The class is offered twice a year in Seattle and, since 1998, twice a year in Bellingham. A total of 150 nurses have now completed the class. This may seem like a small number, but our data reveals that 95 percent of these nurses have supportive and viable programs in their churches. Given the fact that Washington is the least-churched state in the union, this is indeed a blessing!

As a novice teacher, it was by faith alone that I accepted an invitation to facilitate a parish nursing class for the Free Methodist Women's Ministries in June 1995. Now I have done three for them. Since then, I have been invited to facilitate classes in San Diego, Los Angeles, and Kailua, Hawaii. God provides wonderful guest faculty, dedicated participants, and terrific examples of how His people work together to blend faith and health in their communities.

Since 1993, our small interest group of nurses has grown to become a 501(c)3 tax-exempt nonprofit corporation, Puget Sound Parish Nurse Ministries, with a ten-member Board of Directors. We publish a quarterly newsletter, hold two annual continuing education conferences a year, and offer parish nurse professional development meetings in four different locations around Puget Sound. Many members, parish nurses, and supporters now speak publicly within their denominations about parish nursing at annual conferences and other churches, mentor nursing students interested in parish nursing, and conduct research projects, write grants, and publish articles about parish nursing in local newspapers.

There is no greater honor than having women and men from multiple denominations come together to discover that not only do they have much more in common than they have differences, but that God is really in *all* those churches, and that they can laugh, cry, and pray together and become one in God. Through parish nursing and Health Ministries Association involvement and membership, I have had the privilege of meeting many people across the United States who are committed to the faith and health movement, to restoring the church's mission of healing. I am honored to be one small part of this movement.

The Puget Sound Nursing Ministry recently was absorbed into the Northwest Parish Nurse Ministries, and Carol Story has moved into a different phase in her life. She still supports the ministry but has relocated to Arizona to spend time with her mother. She assisted with the establishment of the parish nurse ministry in Bellingham, Washington (see Chapter 8, Reverend Richard Cathell). Carol's influence will not soon be forgotten.

Northwest Parish Nurse Ministries

The last story of this chapter focuses on the Northwest Parish Nurse Ministries (NPNM). Probably the largest network of faith community/parish nurses in the United States, it spans seven states, and offers 135 trainings to over two thousand nurses![8] In

2009 when Carol Story retired as the leader of Puget Sound Nursing Ministry, the leadership of that group asked the NPNM if they could be absorbed into the larger group, adding five hundred additional faith community/parish nurses, plus health ministers to the NPNM roster. In 2005, Annette Stixrud retired from the leadership role in NPNM. Annette had served tirelessly, first as a part-time interim coordinator, from November 1991 to March 1992, then as director of education, and finally as executive director over the course of fourteen years. It is noteworthy that when Annette retired the board separated Annette's responsibilities into two positions—executive director, assumed by Reverend Bruce Strade, and director of education, assumed by Debbie Waring. The history of this network is a fascinating read!

Reverend Bruce Strade, executive director of Northwest Parish Nurse Ministries, agreed to be interviewed and provided the history of the organization, as well as an overview of their programs and accomplishments. A brief summary of the organization's 2009 accomplishments includes:

- Saved millions of dollars in health care costs by promoting prevention and healthy living to at least eighty thousand people in the Northwest and logged well over half a million miles in walking programs.

- Trained sixty-two people as faith community nurses/health ministers in classes held in Portland, Hillsboro, and Bend, Oregon; Tacoma, Washington; and Anchorage, Alaska (totaling well over two thousand since 1992).

- Supported and nurtured over six hundred faith community nurses/health ministers in seven states as they provided a range of services that included blood pressure clinics, health fairs, health classes, walking programs, health counseling, advocacy, home and hospital visits, and countless referrals.

- Provided twelve Living Well with Chronic Conditions workshops in Oregon and Washington for 116 people suffering from one or more chronic illnesses.

- Offered sixteen Powerful Tools for Caregivers classes to 164 family caregivers and trained ten additional class leaders.

- Hosted four regional retreats in Oregon and Washington on The Gift Within: Nurturing and Sustaining a Compassionate Heart, with over 100 in attendance.

- Organized the fourth annual Humor and Health Fest, attracting over 255 people with Jenny Herrick, motivational speaker, author, clown, and nurse, as the featured speaker.

God certainly does prepare those He calls. He scatters seeds and brings forth a harvest that is beyond our imaginings. He has ordained faith community/parish nursing as a ministry and He will continue to orchestrate its development and dissemination throughout the world. The varieties that exist in parish nurse preparation are a true reflection of the richness and diversity that exists within the nursing profession, within the church, and within our world. The journey may indeed lead to the same destination, but there are many alternate routes for the trip.

6. Foundation and Models of Parish Nursing

Therefore everyone who hears these words of mine and puts them into practice is like a wise man who built his house on a rock. The rain came down, the streams rose, and the winds blew and beat against the house; yet it did not fall, because it had its foundation on the rock. But everyone who hears these words of mine and does not put them into practice is like a foolish man who built his house on sand. The rain came down, the streams rose, and the winds blew and beat against the house, and it fell with a great crash.

—Matthew 7:24–27[1]

Any homebuilder knows the importance of starting with a good foundation, or base. In fact, a firm footing is necessary not only for building structures, but also for building character, knowledge, and skills. The foundation has to be solid and it has to be deep enough to support whatever is built or developed on top of it. Likewise, a sound foundation is essential to the practice of the individual parish nurse and for the specialty of parish nursing as well.

In addition to a firm base, blueprints or models aid in new construction. No contractor would begin work on a house or an office building without a plan to follow. The blueprint identifies the design elements and the major aspects of the structure, and illustrates how these elements relate to one another and fit together. A nursing model is very similar to that, in that major concepts are identified and defined and the model illustrates how the concepts work together to produce a coherent whole.

When parish nursing first began, with the vision of Reverend

Granger Westberg, it was well-rooted within the Christian theology of health, healing, and wholeness. Westberg believed in the concept of *shalom*—the Hebrew word for "peace," which also encompasses the sense of "wholeness" and "completeness"—meaning that a person's health was much more than physical well-being or the absence of illness. Westberg viewed the individual as an integrated whole, created to live in harmony with God, self, others, and the environment. This concept of wholeness involves freedom from physical ailments, but so much more. It involves reconciliation with God, being able to give and receive forgiveness, loving and being loved, believing that one's life has purpose and meaning, and experiencing a sense of joy and hope.[2] This is a concept of health and wholeness that goes beyond what medicine alone can offer. Rather, this concept of health and wholeness is what Reverend Westberg believed the parish nurse could facilitate by linking the secular world of high technology and medical interventions with the sacred world of God, prayer, church, and community. These beliefs regarding health and wholeness, and the role of the parish nurse, formed the foundation upon which the first faith community/parish nurses practiced. This model, based on a groundwork of Christian beliefs, was linked to an organizational structure willing to support and extend the model.

The concept of the parish nurse was initiated as a result of a partnership between six churches in the Chicago area and Lutheran General Hospital. As noted in Chapter 5, the hospital supported the original six faith community/parish nurses by paying 75 percent of each nurse's half-time salary; each church supplied the remaining 25 percent of the salary. With each successive year, the hospital decreased its financial support by 25 percent, while the churches increased their financial commitment by 25 percent so that by the fourth year the churches were fully supporting the salaries of the faith community/ parish nurses. As Lutheran General decreased its financial support to the original six churches, that money was freed up to be used to initiate parish nurse positions in other congregations. The partnership between the churches and Lutheran General extended beyond just financial support to include resources for the ongoing development and continuing education of the nurses with half-day weekly supervision sessions held at the hospital. Reverend Westberg provided the supervision, along with the hospital chaplains, a nurse from the hospital teaching program, and a doctor in family medicine.[3]

Granger Westberg envisioned a model of parish nursing that referred to the parish nurse as a "minister of health." He described four major functions of the parish nurse's role: (1) health educator, (2) personal health counselor, (3) trainer of volunteers, and (4) organizer of support groups.[4]

As the idea of parish nursing took hold across the country, it initially remained rooted in a Christian theology of wholeness and used the model outlined by Reverend Westberg. However, over time the organizational structure began to change. Not every parish nurse started her ministry work within a congregation in a salaried position; not every parish nurse received the clinical support provided by Lutheran General Hospital under the guidance of Reverend Granger Westberg. Today, almost three decades after Reverend Westberg worked with the original faith community/parish nurses, the foundation is also changing. Not every parish nurse position is based on Christian theology; parish nursing has become not just interdenominational but also interfaith in scope, with faith community/parish nurses functioning within churches, synagogues, and mosques. In fact, the term *parish nurse* has now been changed to *faith community nurse* in recognition of the broad reach of this specialty beyond the walls of Christian congregations and in accordance with the 2005 *Scope and Standards of Parish Nursing Practice*.[5] In Chapter 5 we heard from Rosemarie Matheus, who stated that although she taught over sixteen hundred faith community/parish nurses, primarily from a Christian perspective, she found it easy to link Old Testament to New Testament teachings in order to demonstrate to Jewish and Muslim nurses that the foundation of parish nursing was rooted in scripture that they accepted and understood. According to Karen Perkin,[6] faith community/parish nursing is consistent with the mission of Jewish-based health care institutions that also have a belief in wholistic health and an obligation to care for those in need.

For instance, Linda Weinberg's story provides an example of how parish nursing is adapted within a Jewish tradition. In a 2001 article published in the *Philadelphia Inquirer*, the health ministry of Linda Weinberg[7] was described. Linda is one of an increasing number of faith community nurses serving Jewish communities across the country. Linda was trained in the Christian model of parish nursing at Villanova University. She then approached the Board of Rabbis about offering her services to synagogues. The only synagogue interested in her services was her own congregation, B'nai Jacob in Phoenixville, Pennsylvania. Linda recruited a group of four volunteer nurses who already worked in conjunction with faith community/parish nurses at a nearby Catholic parish, St. Ann's. In addition to her work with the synagogue, Linda served as the FCN for a project sponsored by the Pew Charitable Trusts. In this role she served people of all faiths, bringing a "Jewish bent" to her ministry. She worked in partnership with a Jewish community chaplain and social worker who made occasional visits. According to Linda, "We are packaged as a bundle with the nurse as the glue in the middle." They visit fourteen area boardinghouses and minister to individuals who are damaged both physically and spiritually. Contrasted with the nurses' stories appearing in Chapter 1 of this book, Linda describes her call in a very different manner.

I don't have the idea of a higher power who is into everyone's lives, but I do think someone's pulling the strings to make me do this. If you ask, "Do I have a Jewish calling to do this?" I say, "Yes I do."

Different Models of Parish Nursing

As noted above, parish nursing today is not a homogeneous specialty. However, when asked to describe the model that they operate under, most nurses who shared their stories for this book responded to that question in terms of whether they were in a paid or unpaid position. Those who were in coordinator positions were paid and those who served an individual faith community were not paid. There are other features that distinguish one model of practice from another.

In the early days of parish nursing, models like the Miller Model of Parish Nursing focused on the practice of the individual nurse within a congregation. As faith community/parish nursing continues to evolve in depth and sophistication, so too are the models that depict the practice. For instance, the model developed by Koenig and Lawson,[8] and referred to in Chapter 2, illustrates the complexity of the parish nurse's pivotal role as she links the secular system of the health care community with the sacred system of the congregation. Many of the nurses who responded to our request for stories for this current edition made reference to practicing according to the Koenig and Lawson model. Sybil Smith[9] makes another distinction among different models based on the underlying philosophy. Each of these models is reviewed below.

Paid versus Unpaid

Across the country the majority of faith community/parish nurses are unpaid for their church-based clinical work. This is also true of the majority of the faith community/parish nurses who responded to our questionnaire. Those who are in paid positions are generally in coordinator roles, either overseeing a large number of volunteers within their own congregations or in a hospital-based coordinator role overseeing a congregational network. The story of Linda Scott, a nurse educator at Concordia College in Moorhead, Minnesota, is a typical one.

The model I started at First Lutheran Church in Brookings, South Dakota, was a volunteer model because my congregation was struggling to stay within budget. I knew that there was no money to add expenses for a new program and a volunteer model would allow us to get started. I proposed that we operate under a volunteer model for two years, and then reevaluate. I hoped to seek funding through a grant. Also, I hoped that the congregation would recognize the program's worth and be willing to budget at least a small portion toward materials and expenses.

My congregation of about two thousand did reimburse me for the cost of the Parish Nurse Preparation course and for some of the supplies that we needed for our annual health fair. Also, the congregation made space available and office supplies for a little office in the "mother's cry room." This "cry room" had a restroom, a space for infants and small children, and a window to the sanctuary. It worked well as a space to conduct our Sunday morning blood pressure screenings between services because it was an existing space that lent itself to multipurpose use. The other kind of support I received was encouragement from the pastors and church council for whatever health-related activities I had time to pursue.

I was the coordinator of this unpaid model. There were three to four RNs with current licenses who worked with me. In addition, I had the support of two retired RNs and two to three other women who were interested in serving as health volunteers. We operated under this model from August 1993 through May 1998. At that time, I moved away to another state. We must have gained the trust of the congregation, though, because after I left an arrangement was worked out with the hospital and a new PN was hired.

As this current edition of *Parish Nursing* was being prepared, Linda was contacted for an update on her role within this specialty.

I'm an unpaid PN at my church and practice parish nursing minimally. My greatest connection to parish nursing now is through my faculty role at Concordia College, where our nursing students work with the Faithfully Fit Forever program at my church. As you probably know, typically that program is geared toward older adults to keep them active physically, mentally, and spiritually, but one of my colleagues modified and initiated the program for children and now I carry it out through the Community Health Nursing course that I teach.

Many of the faith community/parish nurses who shared their stories with us communicated a similar sentiment as Linda Whitesell, a faith community/parish nurse with Prince of Peace Lutheran Church in Everett, Washington, who participated in the first edition of the book.

I have been a parish nurse since 1998 and now feel more competent in my role as I have become more familiar with the needs of my congregants. They too have learned to trust my judgment and acknowledge my skills regarding wellness and health-related issues. My status remains as a volunteer. I feel that it is my special contribution to my congregation. I do not think I would take a salary even if it was offered.

Some faith community/parish nurses wore more than one hat. For instance, Kris Wisnefske, RN, MSN, is both a faith community/ parish nurse and a parish nurse-coordinator. Currently, she serves as a parish nurse for her Catholic church—this is a volunteer position; however, in the past this has been a paid position. She works about fifteen to twenty hours per month at her church. Since January 2002, Kris has also served as the parish nurse coordinator through Monroe Clinic in Monroe, Wisconsin. Kris is also the chair of the Wisconsin Parish Nurse Coalition (WPNC), which is a special interest group of the WNA (Wisconsin Nurses Association).

Rosemarie Matheus (see Chapter 5), one of the pioneers in parish nurse preparation and the director of the Parish Nurse Institute at Marquette University School of Nursing, was asked about models of parish nursing and she also responded regarding whether or not the nurse is paid or not. Rosemarie states:

When I was teaching students who were enrolled in my Parish Nurse Preparation course, I encouraged them to avoid the term volunteer model. When people are describing a volunteer model, there is frequently a negative connotation to "just being a volunteer." I always suggested that nurses should make the distinction between paid and unpaid with the hope that if they are in an unpaid position there is always the possibility that it will become a paid position.

I definitely have a bias for the paid model. I have worked with both of these models and find that there are problems with the unpaid model, especially if a hospital is supporting it. There is nothing beyond the spirit of the individual nurse that compels the nurse to put in a certain number of hours, to maintain a documentation system, or to meet any of the hospital's quality standards. If a hospital system is supporting an unpaid parish nurse program under the umbrella of the hospital, it raises serious ethical questions.

I have heard people say that the church must make a financial contribution to the salary of the parish nurse. Although I believe the parish nurse should be paid, the salary can come from either the church, the hospital, or from both. I have observed quite a few situations where the church has paid nothing and this did not seem to influence whether or not the congregation respected the contributions of the parish nurse or even if the role of the parish nurse was fully integrated into the ministry program of the congregation.

I suggested to my students that if their church says that it cannot "afford" a parish nurse, they enter into a covenant with the congregation. They offer to work for nine to twelve months in a pilot role. At the end of the pilot program, the church then reevaluates the value of the parish nurse's contributions. If the church believes that the parish nurse is making important contributions, then the contract is rewritten and a salary is agreed upon. Initially, the salary may not be what the nurse might receive in the open market, but it is a start. I have found that in 90 percent of these situations, churches are willing to pay the nurse.[10]

Model Depicting Individual Parish Nurse Function

There are a number of good examples of these types of models.[11] One of the earliest was created by Dr. Linda Miller as part of her doctoral dissertation and was published in the winter 1997 issue of JCN.[12] Miller describes the underlying worldview of the Miller Model of Parish Nursing as evangelical Christian. She presents her model in the form of three stained-glass windows, each illustrating a different aspect of parish nursing. The first stained-glass window depicts the concepts central to all nursing practice—the nurse (the parish nurse); health (presented in terms of the Christian tradition of shalom, or wholeness); the context of care (the church); and the person receiving care (the congregant). In the center of the first stained-glass window is the concept of the triune God—the Father,

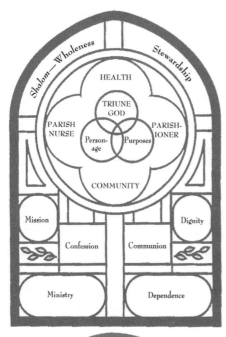

Box 6.1 Components and major concepts of the model. Used with permission by Lynda W. Miller, RN, PhD. First appeared in *Journal of Christian Nursing*, Winter 1997, 17–20.

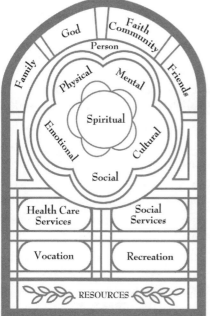

Box 6.2 Aspects of the whole person (spiritual, physical, mental, emotional, social, cultural) and health-promoting resources of the person. First appeared in *Journal of Christian Nursing*, Winter 1997, 17–20.

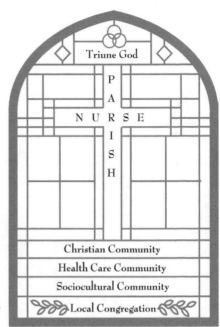

Box 6.3 Contexts of the parish nurse role. First appeared in *Journal of Christian Nursing*, Winter 1997, 17–20.

the Son, and the Holy Spirit. This theological concept of the triune God, or the trinity, is a core tenet of the Christian faith, affirmed for over twenty centuries of church history and serving as a unifying concept for Christians, regardless of their cultural or denominational differences.

The second stained-glass window depicts the complex and interconnected dimensions of the person and how that person relates to health-promoting resources, such as God, family, the faith community, friends, health care and social services, vocation, and recreation. In the third stained-glass window, Miller shows the many contexts of the parish nurse role, including the Christian, health care, and sociocultural communities, as well as the local congregation. The figures for the Miller Model of Parish Nursing are included in Box 6.1–6.3.

The Parish Nurse as Link Between Sacred and Secular

A model developed by Koenig and Lawson[13] and shown in Box 6.4 focuses on the functions of the parish nurse and clearly demonstrates the vital role that the parish nurse fulfills as the link between the church community and the health care community.

This model (also referred to in Chapter 2) represents an evolutionary view of the significance of parish nursing to the health care system as we continue to move into the twenty-first century. Dr. Harold G. Koenig, one of the authors of this book, believes that faith community/ parish nurses will play an increasingly critical role in the provision of health care in the future. As the number of aged Americans expands and their needs for comprehensive health care increase, the capacity of the health care system to provide this care will shrink. If today's

Functions of the Parish Nurse

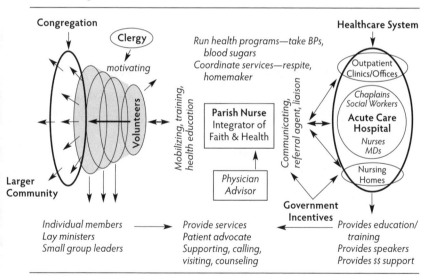

Box 6.4 Adapted from Koenig, H. G., & Lawson, D. M. (2004). *Faith in the future: Healthcare, aging, and the role of religion.* Philadelphia: Templeton Foundation Press.

resources seem barely adequate, tomorrow's may seem scarce to non-existent when it comes to long-term comprehensive care. The parish nurse provides a solution to this dilemma of shrinking resources in the face of expanding needs. Through the nurse's ability to train and mobilize volunteers within the church community, faith community/parish nurses can serve as care extenders when the traditional health care system is stretched to the breaking point. Through her functions as educator and counselor, the parish nurse motivates and equips church volunteers to carry out preventive care activities, provide respite for overburdened families and caregivers, offer spiritual support, and assist in the monitoring and management of chronic illnesses, again decreasing the burden on the traditional health care system. This model is particularly important in congregations that contain many people with health problems needing care. If the parish nurse tried to meet all these preventive, spiritual, and health care needs herself, she would rapidly become overwhelmed and burned out; hence the emphasis on being a trainer and motivator of volunteers. Through her role as an integrator of faith and health, the parish nurse draws the power of belief, prayer, ritual, and community into the equation of health and healing.

Faith Community/Parish Nurse as Servant Leader

In a new book, titled *Servant Leadership in Nursing: Spirituality and Practice in Contemporary Health Care*, to be published in 2010, Sister Mary Elizabeth O'Brien[14] writes about the importance of being a servant first. This model comes directly from the teachings and example of Jesus, who told His followers:

You know that the rulers of the Gentiles lord it over them, and their high officials exercise authority over them. Not so with you. Instead, whoever wants to become great among you must be your servant, and whoever wants to be first must be your slave—just as the Son of Man did not come to be served, but to serve, and to give his life as a ransom for many. (Matthew 20:25–28)

Robert K. Greenleaf, in his classic essay "The Servant as Leader," described the servant-leader in this manner:

The servant-leader is servant first . . . It begins with the natural feeling that one wants to serve, to serve first. Then conscious choice brings one to aspire to lead. That person is sharply different from one who is leader first, perhaps because of the need to assuage an unusual power drive or to acquire material possessions. . . . The leader-first and the servant-first are two extreme types. Between them there are shadings and blends that are part of the infinite variety of human nature.

The difference manifests itself in the care taken by the servant-first to make sure that other people's highest-priority needs are being served. The best test, and a difficult one to administer, is this: Do those served grow as persons? Do they, while being served, become healthier, wiser, freer, more autonomous, more likely themselves to become servants? And, what is the effect on the least privileged in society? Will they benefit or at least not be further deprived?[15]

Kris Wisnefske and Tammy Koenecke, both faith community/ parish nurse-coordinators in Wisconsin, gave a presentation titled Integration of Servant Leadership Characteristics in Parish Nurse Practice. Their presentation reviewed the characteristics of a servant-leader and made the natural connection to parish nursing. Kris and Tammy provided many examples of servant-leaders, including Jesus, Mother Teresa, Mahatma Gandhi, Martin Luther King Jr., and Dorothy Day. Their presentation challenged attendees to assess their current leadership styles and to ask themselves whether they were called to be servant-leaders. The next steps involved learning more about what this concept means; certainly studying the stories of the notable servant-leaders is an excellent place to begin. In addition, the faith community/parish nurse needs to serve as a role model for others by modeling the characteristics of servant-leadership, including excellent listening skills, empathy, healing, awareness, persuasion, the ability to conceptualize, foresight, stewardship, and commitment to the growth of others as well as community. Sounds like servant-leadership is a perfect fit for faith community/parish nursing!

Access, Marketplaces, and Mission/Ministry Models

The last types of models that we examine in this chapter are delineated by Sybil Smith.[16] Smith believes that as parish nursing moves more into the mainstream of health care, it begins to take on a different character. Understanding the underlying philosophy behind various parish nursing models helps church leaders to choose a model that is congruent with their ministry goals. Smith describes three types of models: access, market, and ministry. Access models are driven by a belief that equal access to health care is a right for all. Although access models are inherently political in nature, this does not preclude the role of faith. However, the underpinning for the access model is not a faith-based belief in shalom, but rather theories of advocacy, poverty, justice, and empowerment. These theories are often tied to philosophies of public health science and community health. Parish nursing becomes the means to increase access to health care for those for whom the door to health care is often closed. The integration of faith, although possible, is not the focus of such models. In the story of Linda Weinberg, presented earlier in this chapter, we saw an example of an access model in her work with the fourteen boardinghouses in the Philadelphia area and supported by the Pew Charitable Trusts.

The *marketplace models* are tied in some way to a health care system. In this model, parish nursing is operated through home care, case management, community outreach, marketing and business-development departments, and other departments within a health care system. Marketplace models are driven by economic values and offer a commodity to a congregation. Sometimes the parish nurse program is used as a marketing or public relations tool, in hopes of increasing the market share of the health care system that is served by the parish nurse. The nurse may or may not be a member of the congregation served, which means that she may or may not have a vested interest in the welfare of the community as a member as well as a committed believer. The church facility is the site for delivering health services. Inreach programs for church members, as well as outreach programs to the underserved in neighboring communities, are provided through the marketplace model. However, whatever is provided in some way benefits the bottom line of the health care system. Although the term *parish nurse* is used, it is inappropriate in this context, because the nurse's main efforts are not on behalf of the congregation but rather the health care system. Sometimes the nurse employed by a marketplace model experiences real values conflict when her motivation of ministry clashes with her employer's motivation of profit.

Mission/Ministry Models

The last type of model to be discussed is the *mission/ministry model*. In this model the nurse can be either a paid or an unpaid staff member on the ministry team of the church. The nurse who functions in a mission/ministry role has experienced "God's call" to this ministry. The focus is less on the role of the nurse but more on the people served. Nurses feel called to be stewards of their faith and in responding to this call they find their lives infused with meaning and purpose. The mission of the parish nurse is to be an integrator of faith and health and, in doing so, to help church members to endure the spiritual, emotional, and physical challenges of life that come to each of us. This is the model represented by most of the stories of nurses told throughout this book. These nurses join with their fellow parishioners, coming together in worship and prayer to share in the healing ministry of their God and their church community.

Many parish nursing programs represent a blend of these various models. As we look at faith community/parish nursing, we see a living and growing specialty. The one constant that exists in anything that lives and grows—whether it is a person, a plant, an idea, a system, or an organization—is change. We can expect change to continue within faith community/parish nursing as it responds to various calls: the call of God, the call of the health care system, the call of the individual nurse-practitioner, and the call of the person served by this unique ministry. In the next chapter we hear nurses tell us the step-by-step process of starting a parish nurse program and the resources that helped them do so.

7. Establishing a Faith Community/ Parish Nurse Program

There is an old saying, "Don't go where the path leads, go where there is no path and leave a trail."[1] Many faith community/parish nurses testify to the truth of this saying as they share their stories of beginning faith community/parish nurse programs in their own congregations. The developmental process and growing pains of such a ministry are unique to each nurse and congregation. Yet there are similar steps that many nurses identify that might facilitate the passage for others.

In this chapter we examine some general steps for initiating a faith community/parish nursing program. We then turn our attention to the stories of nurses as they embarked on this journey, often without a clear path to pursue but leaving a valuable trail behind for others to follow. Last, we return to faith community/parish nurses themselves, who provide advice to others interested in starting on a similar path.

Beginning Steps

In his book The Parish Nurse, Reverend Granger Westberg[2] identified six steps for starting a faith community/parish nurse program, including:

1. Learn as much as possible.
2. Include the pastor and other church leaders in the initial dialogue.
3. Form a health committee.

4. Try to establish a link with a hospital.

5. Select and orient a nurse.

6. Begin the program.

Judith Shelly, a former parish nurse in Obelisk, Pennsylvania, and former editor of the *Journal of Christian Nursing*, expands on these steps with the following suggestions:

1. The nurse who leads the program needs a vision for health ministry.

2. A mission statement is essential to effectively communicate the purpose and benefits of parish nursing to the governing body of the church as well as to the congregation at large.

3. Initial funding must be budgeted to cover the start-up costs of supplies, education, and congregational programs.

4. Personal malpractice insurance is essential for individual faith community/parish nurses.

5. The church needs to obtain malpractice insurance covering this program; this can be usually added as a rider to the church's property insurance for a nominal amount.

St. Joseph's Hospital Health Center's Congregational Health Program in Syracuse, New York, under the leadership of Marianne Parker, developed useful resources to support the steps identified by Westberg and Shelly. These resources provide detailed samples and explanations of each of the steps to guide the development of a faith community/parish nurse/health ministry program. The Informational Packet, referred to in Box 7.1, educates the reader about health ministry and parish nursing; the values of these programs; the history of faith community/parish nursing; the scope of services; and the steps to take in starting a health ministry/faith community/parish nurse program. The Policy and Forms Informational Guide, referred to in Box 7.2, provides samples of documents, such as mission statements and bulletin/newsletter blurbs, inviting participation in health ministry.

St. Joseph's Hospital Health Center's Mission

1. Congregational Health Program Purpose
2. Taking a Look at the Public and Private Health Issues
3. Why Call upon the Faith Community?
4. St. Joseph's Hospital Health Center (SJHHC) Congregational Health Program
   a. Parish Nursing
   b. Congregational Health Ministry
   c. Education and Training
   d. Wellness Programming
   e. Agency Liaison
5. What are the qualifications to become a faith community/parish nurse?
6. What are the common models for faith community/parish nursing/ health ministry?
7. Do faith community/parish nurses have to document?
8. History of Parish Nursing
9. Defining Parish Nursing: What is the role of a faith community/ parish nurse?
10. Steps in establishing a faith community/parish nursing/health ministry program
11. Defining Congregational Health Ministry
12. How do we implement a health ministry/faith community/parish nurse program?
13. Program Participation: SJHHC's Congregational Health Programs Coordinator
14. Program Participation: The Local Faith Community
15. Wellness Programming
16. Agency Liaison
17. Education and Training

Box 7.1 (cont.)

18. Resource Library
19. Health Fair Supplies
20. Additional Resources
    a. Policy and Forms Information Guide
    b. Health Fair Planning Guide
    c. Growth and Development Guide
    d. ANA Continuing Education Take-Home Articles
    e. SJHHC School of Nursing Library—available to faith community/
       parish nurses in SJHHC Congregational Health Program
21. Bibliography

Box 7.2 Policy and Forms Informational Guide. Used with permission of St. Joseph's Hospital Health Center's Congregation Health Program.

1. Mission Statement
2. Sample Communication with Your Congregation
3. Job Description—Coordinator
4. Job Description—Faith Community/Parish Nurse
5. Job Description—Health Cabinet
6. Confidentiality Recommendation—Mandatory Reporting of Abuse
7. Visitation Recommendation
8. Blood Pressure Consent/Documentation
9. Blood Pressure Booklet Master
10. Annual Planning Outline
11. Monthly Summary
12. Annual Evaluation
13. Health Ministry Survey

When we asked nurses to share their stories, several of the questions we posed to them included the following:

- How did you get started?
- What were your experiences convincing your parish/congregation that parish nursing was a valuable addition to the church's ministry?
- How did you introduce the concept to the church at large?
- What type of reception did you receive?

Getting Started: Pray

Almost unanimously, nurses told us that one of the first steps, and one that they revisit throughout their journeys, is the need for prayer. In addition to praying, Dr. Sagrid E. Edman, RN, PhD, the former Nursing Department chair at Bethel College in St. Paul, Minnesota, suggests that nurses who are considering entering a health ministry as a faith community/parish nurse reflect on the following issues:

- Ask yourself whether or not you have the spiritual resources to continuously share with others.
- Can you give up the typical nurse role of "fixer of every situation"?
- Are you a team player? Loners don't make good faith community/parish nurses, nor do they facilitate a successful congregational health ministry.
- Are you able to be creative and think outside the usual clinical or hospital "box"?
- Are you someone church members will be able to trust? A congregation is not a hospital system with patients as a captive audience. Congregants will not consult with someone they do not trust.

Another common start-up issue is preparation. The nurses who responded to our questionnaire reported that they sought out some sort of faith community/parish nurse preparation. This preparation varied from a series of one-day workshops to a semester-long course offered through a seminary or a university setting. Many mentioned attending one of the courses referred to in Chapter 5. Another frequent comment focused on whether or not the particular preparation had been endorsed by the International Parish Nurse Resource Center.

Linda Scott reports,

In 1993, I took the basic Faith Community/Parish Nurse Preparation class through Concordia College at Moorhead, Minnesota. The course consisted of four parts: (1) the faith community/parish nurse role: integrating faith and health issues; (2) wholistic health and wellness concepts for the faith community/parish nurse; (3) the faith community/parish nurse as a personal health counselor and advocate; and (4) the faith community/parish nurse working with people across the life span. Since there were so few faith community/parish nurses practicing at this time, there was no clinical component for "shadowing" of a faith community/ parish nurse—we just had to visualize what the role would look like. The program that I attended was later endorsed by the International Parish Nurse Resource Center but with additional classes required. I went back to Concordia to complete those classes.

Dr. Sagrid E. Edman enrolled in the course taught by Rosemarie Matheus at Marquette. This course was also endorsed by the International Parish Nurse Resource Center.

The course at Marquette gave us almost more than we could handle, in terms of bibliographies, journal articles, health-related material, and free sources of wellness pamphlets and teaching materials. I wanted to take the course from Rosemarie. She has a very global perspective on parish nursing. Taking this course was where I experienced a "call" to become a faith community/parish nurse. Everything about the ministry of parish nursing fit what I felt God wanted me to do in my retirement. I didn't really learn much that was new, but the course put nursing in the perspective and context of the congregation and gave me a good feel for the roles and boundaries of parish nursing. It fit with my years as a nursing educator.

It fit with what I think nursing is all about—a compassionate, caring, and healing ministry.

Convincing the Church Leadership

A successful faith community/parish nurse program requires the full support of the pastor and other church leaders. Some of the nurses reported that the idea originated with the pastor, who convinced the church leadership; other nurses needed to first convince the pastor before moving on with program development, shares Carole Kornelis, a faith community/parish nurse for First Reformed Church in Lynden, Washington:

Our pastor of older adults, Pastor Eric, brought the concept of parish nursing to the Ministry Team. He had heard about parish nursing at a conference in the Midwest and was excited about the prospect of bringing parish nursing into our church family. He called a meeting with the nurses of the congregation and others who might be interested. He invited Carol Story, the director of Puget Sound Parish Nurse Ministries, to speak and showed a short video, titled "An Introduction to Health Ministry and Parish Nursing: The Healing Team," which portrayed what parish nursing was all about and how useful it was to congregations. The idea was enthusiastically accepted and we were off and running.

The Parish Nurse Commission of the Northwest Conference of the Evangelical Covenant Church serves Minnesota, Wisconsin, Iowa, and South Dakota. This group, which has been instrumental in moving parish nursing forward in these states, had an interesting start. Sagrid Edman tells the story.

Our district superintendent's wife had a vision for parish nursing for several years. It began when her husband was a pastor at one of our local Minnesota churches. When he became superintendent, she began pestering him about helping churches get started with a faith community/ parish nurse ministry. The way to do that, he said, was to collect a group of faith community/parish nurses, write a proposal for support and funding, and present it to the Conference Board that he reports to. So that's what she did in the fall of 1997. She called together a group of five, all of whom had either taken the Faith Community/Parish Nursing course or were going to. Several were already in faith community/parish nurse positions in their churches. We collaborated on writing a proposal and presented it to the board. It was accepted with strong support. The proposal was for a matching grant to help the churches start the ministry. The funding was to support a preparation course for faith community/parish nursing, plus budget for one-time start-up office equipment and supplies for a total of $1,400. Participating churches had to submit a budget showing their half of the funding.

We wrote to all the churches with information about the funding, developed a brochure, included an information sheet and articles about faith community/parish nurse ministry, and offered to meet with the appropriate committee, board, or group at each church to explain what a faith community/parish nursing program was all about. Then the task force fanned out and met with churches, as we were requested. So it began, one church at a time.

The churches were all receptive, but not all could see the importance of the ministry. Those who were less supportive said things like, "We go to the health club every week. Why would we need a faith community/parish nurse?" Or "All our parishioners have their own doctor. Why would we go to a faith community/parish nurse to have our blood pressure taken?" Slowly, the concept has taken hold. Most of the pastors who have a faith community/parish nurse say that they do not know what they would do without one.

In 1997 we had five congregations in the conference that had some type of faith community/parish nursing ministry. A few were unofficial and very part-time. Today we have twenty-five to thirty churches in the Northwest Conference with faith community/parish nurse ministries!

Introducing Parish Nursing to the Congregation

The introduction of parish nursing to the congregation usually takes many forms. One of the most powerful is pulpit support, and involves the pastor preaching on the importance of a health ministry to the church. The pastor's support and explanation about the role of a faith community/parish nurse as part of health ministry, the importance of whole-person health, and the fact that the church's mission is not just to preach and teach but to heal as well, gives immeasurable backing to a new faith community/parish nurse and a health ministry. Another approach involves inserting an announcement into the church bulletin or newsletter. A sample is presented in Box 7.3.

Catherine Lomax, a faith community/parish nurse in Paoli, Pennsylvania, spoke to the congregation during all three services. This is what she shared:

As I start my journey to serve you, my prayers are that we can journey together side by side. Parish nursing is an old concept, brought back to meet the needs of today's churches. It involves a wholistic approach, including body, mind, and spirit. We will focus on the close relationship between our faith and our health. With the support of the Health

---

Box 7.3   Adapted from Policy and Forms Informational Guide. Used with permission of St. Joseph's Hospital Health Center's Congregation Health Program.

Sample Bulletin/Newsletter Blurb:
First Presbyterian Church of Chittenango

We are expanding a new ministry to meet the needs of our congregation and community. This health and healing ministry will use the talents of nurses, other health professionals, and laypeople interested in the healing ministry of the church. We are under the supervision of deacons. We need to expand the health cabinet and reach into additional areas of church and community life. There will be an information meeting on [insert date] from 6 to 7 p.m. All interested people are encouraged to attend. For more information call [insert phone number].

Cabinet, we will be doing a parish survey to collect information to assist us in setting up programs regarding health education and illness management, counseling, blood pressure screening, and other health-related issues. I will be visiting those who are sick and shut-in to assess their health needs and to link these members with congregational and community resources. I am looking forward to meeting the volunteers of the church. As a volunteer myself, I find that volunteering provides a way of both giving to others and receiving back. I ask God to put it on your hearts to come and serve Him and to share your gifts with others in the church. I will have office hours and my door will be open to you to discuss whatever concerns you. I am creating a brochure that I will distribute with more information about my role as faith community/parish nurse, my office hours, and telephone numbers to reach me. I look forward to getting to know and meet each of you. Thank you and God bless.

The last way to obtain the congregation's "buy-in" of the faith community/parish nursing program is to talk up the ministry during informal meetings. Personally reaching out to others who have a passion for the healing ministry and inviting their participation is an effective means of increasing grassroots support. Engaging the coordinators and members of the other ministries within the church strengthens collaboration and expands the scope of the services that the nurse can access. Although the list of ministries varies from congregation to congregation, the following are possible considerations for faith community/parish nurse outreach:

• the religious school

• deacons

• the parish or church council

• Eucharistic ministers

• community outreach

• the food pantry

• the social ministry

- human development
- Stephen ministers
- life teams
- the caregiver committee
- the lay pastoral team

The majority of nurses who responded to our questionnaire were welcomed by their congregations. However, some encountered a mixed response. Let's listen to Linda Scott's story.

Presenting the concept of parish nursing to my congregation challenged me in ways I had not expected. I thought every nurse would believe in the philosophy of parish nursing as I did . . . that it was the kind of nursing that we all longed for. But I found that my colleagues and congregational members were either all for the idea or totally against it. There seemed to be no middle ground. Those who opposed the idea voiced concern that parish nursing would threaten the local home health agency. Others were concerned about the liability of a nurse practicing in the church. Some of the greatest advocates for parish nursing believed, as I did, that parish nursing could respond to their calling to care rather than just the need for employment.

Donna Benning, a faith community/parish nurse in Bellingham, Washington, describes her initial reception as one of "blank stares."

What turned the tide for me was actually providing care for a church member and then conducting the memorial service when he died. When the congregants began to see my role in action, it made a huge difference in my acceptance within the church. Another important element in my acceptance was when I started to put together small teams to assist the ill with yardwork and housekeeping chores.

Advice to Other Faith Community/Parish Nurses

Nurses shared the following advice with others interested in parish nursing:

- Pray.

- Take a faith community/parish nurse course that is recommended by its participants.

- Read everything you can on faith community/parish nursing.

- Attend at least one Westberg Symposium.

- Spend some time with a faith community/parish nurse as she "lives out" her role.

- Start small and build a foundation of acceptance.

- Build relationships—with individual church members, with existing ministries within the church, and with community resources.

- Set reasonable goals.

- Enjoy the freedom of being able to integrate your faith into your practice.

- Be strong and comfortable in your own faith.

- Be open to various forms of prayer and spirituality.

- Network with other faith community/parish nurses so you don't feel like you are "out there by yourself."

- Maintain balance in your own life. Be able to say "no," lean on others, and set appropriate professional and personal boundaries.

Sometimes a journey is easy and uneventful; other times it is halting, slow, and uncertain. It helps to have a map—it is reassuring to know the terrain. It also helps to know that someone has successfully completed this same journey before you. And it helps to know that God travels with you.

Faith community/parish nurses share the map with each other. They prepare each other for the terrain. Many are far along on the journey and they beckon others to join them. All of them know that God goes before and with them.

In the next chapter we look forward to possibilities as the journey of parish nursing continues.

8. Looking to the Future
The Next Generation of Parish Nursing

Most of us spend time musing about what we will do tomorrow, next week, next year, even five years from now, believing that we can control our destiny. Too often we are painfully confronted with the reality that our sense of control is at best illusory. This, however, does not stop us from forecasting, predicting, and certainly not from dreaming. So we conclude this book about the experiences of parish nurses with a glimpse into what might be—not only for individual parish nurses, but also for this nursing specialty and for the health care system that stands to benefit greatly from the contributions of these loving servants of God.

As we spoke to many faith community/parish nurses and read the stories of many others, we were impressed by a number of major changes that have taken place in this specialty. First, the name change is important to note. In 2005 the Health Ministries Association, in conjunction with the American Nurses Association, published *Faith Community Nursing: Scope and Standards of Practice*[1] and adopted the name *faith community nursing* (FCN) in place of *parish nursing* "in order to adopt an all-encompassing title for this specialty."

Second, the specialty is exploding—not only in the number of nurses but also in its international spread. In 2002, when we wrote the first edition of this book, there were approximately five thousand faith community/parish nurses. Today there are at least twelve thousand, and that number continues to grow. Faith community/parish nursing is now practiced in many countries outside the United States.

Its global reach extends to the United Kingdom, Canada, Australia, New Zealand, Israel, Korea, South Africa, and Pakistan.

Another change is the increase in support and involvement of many national and international organizations. In the United States this support comes from such diverse organizations as the following:

- International Parish Nurse Resource Center (IPNRC) (www.parishnurses.org)
- Health Ministries Association (HMA) (www.healthministriesassociation.org)
- Health Ministries Network of Minnesota (www.healthministries .info)
- Northwest Parish Nurse Ministries (www.npnm.org)
- Nurses Christian Fellowship (www.ncf-jcn.org/)

Internationally, the organizations supporting this specialty include the following:

- Anglican Health Care Ministry Cabinet (www.anglicanhealthcareministry.weebly.com)
- Australian Parish Nurse Resource Center (www.apnrc.org)
- Canadian Association for Parish Nursing Ministry (www .capnm.ca)
- Ecumenical Health Care Ministry Council (www.ecumenicalhealthcareministry.weebly.com)
- Interchurch Health Ministries (ICHM) (www.ichm.ca)
- New Zealand Faith Community Nurses Association (www .faithnursing.co.nz)
- Parish Nursing Ministries UK (www.parishnursing.co.uk)

Educational Preparation

Educational preparation has also expanded dramatically. Within the United States, preparation for this specialty can be obtained from the IPNRC and 140 educational partners, including universities, colleges, medical centers, individual hospitals, and seminaries. The preparation has expanded to encompass a range of training options, including the following:

- Basic Preparation Course: Developed to respond to the need for core faith community nurse content.

- Coordinator Preparation Course: Provides material to help the nurse who supervises programs, and works with institutions, agencies, and various faith communities.

- Faculty Preparation Course: Designed to prepare faith community nurses wishing to teach others the Basic Prep Course.

- Supplemental Modules 2005 and Supplemental Modules 2007: Developed for use in faith community nurse continuing education.[2]

There are also post-master's certifications in faith community nursing. For instance, Azusa Pacific University's School of Nursing offers such a program. Duke's Health and Nursing Ministries Program will prepare students to serve as national and international leaders in the development and coordination of congregational and community-based health care programs. Students may enroll in one of three educational programs: master's in church ministries/health and nursing ministries track; master of science in nursing/health with a nursing ministries major; or a joint master's degree in church ministries/master of science in nursing. These three joint programs of study may be taken either full-time or part-time. A post-master's certificate program is also available for the master's-prepared nurse seeking further education in the field of congregation-based health ministry.

Certification as a Specialist in Nursing

There are efforts being made to develop a clinical certification for faith community nurses. The Health Ministries Association, the IPNRC, and the Faith Community Nurse (FCN) Recognition Committee have been working with the American Nurses Credentialing Center (ANCC) to develop a strategy to credential faith community nurses through a web-based portfolio process, rather than a written exam. The portfolio process will offer the FCN candidate an opportunity to show that she has met the standards set forth in the American Nurses Association's 2005 edition of *Faith Community Nursing: Scope and Standards of Nursing Practice*.

Growth of Networks of FCNs

According to Reverend Dr. Deborah Patterson, executive director of the IPNRC, there are over 240 parish nurse coordinators who provide support to networks of individual faith community/parish nurses. This support is in the form of guidance, resources, and education. Generally speaking, the network coordinator's post is a paid position supported by a hospital system and paid from operational funds that are reported to the federal government as community service dollars.[3]

Increase in Research Efforts

Faith community nurses are beginning to validate the impact of their efforts through research. Laura Rydholm,[4] a parish nurse in Minnesota and a true pioneer in the area of faith community/parish nurse outcome studies, has been the principal investigator in several studies. The most recently published of these studies, which came out in 2007, details the use of a documentation system called "DIARY," an acronym for Data, Interpretation, Action, Response, and Yield as part of a larger study launched by the Metropolitan Area Agency on Aging in Minnesota and supported by the Minnesota Department of Human Services and the Medica Foundation—both stakeholders in elder care and illness prevention.

The focus of the larger study was to explore existing faith-based support networks that older adults access informally while at the same time improving communication between faith-based networks and quasi-formal and formal systems of care. The ultimate goal was to make available to elderly caregivers and at-risk older adults supports such as coaches, assistants, and available first responders. The evaluation component of the larger project was the Parish Nurse Effectiveness Study, which was designed to identify concerns regarding limited access to care experienced by older adults, the interventions used by parish nurses to address the concerns of elders, and the cost savings that might result from the interventions of parish nurses.

Parish nurses who participated in the study were given training on the use of the DIARY documentation system. They were paid a $20 stipend for each note submitted to the researchers. Notes were submitted by seventy-five parish nurses; these notes focused on recent elder care experiences, resulting in 1,061 notes in total. All notes were coded and analyzed. Two-thirds of the contributed notes were in a ready-to-quantify format, but the remaining third—the narrative notes—needed to be translated into the DIARY tool.[5] The data were sorted and categorized and the results demonstrated that one-third of the nurses' notes pertained to urgent matters; one-third focused on needs for functional support; and the last third dealt with the need for psychosocial support. Spiritual and psychosocial issues accounted for 40 percent of the concerns of the older adults receiving care from parish nurses; signs and symptoms necessitating care were the focus of 25 percent of the concerns of elders; functional and safety concerns accounted for 14 percent of the total; illness and self-care deficits contributed another 9 percent; depression accounted for 8 percent of these concerns; and detrimental lifestyle habits accounted for 4 percent to the concerns of the older adults.

In addition to the quantitative analysis performed by the researchers, a qualitative analysis was also done. This yielded stories of frail older adults who were ignoring symptoms of serious conditions, such as impending strokes, heart attacks, renal and/or heart failure, respiratory failure, sepsis, falls, nerve damage related to unattended fractures, and medicine toxicity. Symptoms of these serious conditions were usually ignored as a cost-saving measure. If the nurses' evaluations of the effectiveness of their interventions were accurate, the cost savings to Medicare as a result of their efforts were probably in excess of $3 million.

The interventions of the faith community nurses successfully provided a bridge of care to older adults between an informal, faith-based system and the formal, acute care system. With the graying of the baby boomers, this role of the faith community nurse will become even more crucial in containing medical costs for chronic illnesses.

Another important outcome study, published by Brown et al. (2009),[6] also reported on measurable health outcomes demonstrating cost savings to families, communities, and health systems associated with the interventions of FCNs. The three networks of FCNs taking part in this study were able to show more than $600,000 in savings (for calendar year 2008) by preventing acute care visits and extended care placements. Brown et al. (2009) also stated that within the three networks of FCNs participating in this study, 20 percent of the contacts were with people outside their congregations.

A Powerful Story of Change

We have chosen to highlight the following story, which we believe provides a glimpse into the possible future of parish or faith community nursing. This story exemplifies the growth of FCNs, the importance of a network, the vital role of leadership and vision, and the extension of service to communities beyond the walls of the individual faith communities. We learned about this story by speaking with Carole Kornelis, who participated in the first edition of this book, and was gracious enough to share with us her continuing journey as a FCN/PN. She encouraged us to contact Reverend Richard (Dick) Cathell, the administrative liaison for faith community nurses in Bellingham, Washington. Carole told us, "Dick is a great resource. He is our parish nurse administrative liaison and has great ideas and connections within the hospital and community. Because of his enthusiasm and interest, he has taken our coalition of parish nurses and given us a new beginning and fresh ideas."

We were so intrigued that we immediately contacted the reverend and asked if he would share his story with us. We spent an hour and a half on the telephone, feverishly writing what Dick so generously shared. Carole was right! His ideas are exciting and fresh, and suggest a model for faith community nursing that not only could be adopted in other areas of the country but could be effective in meeting the health care needs of the local community beyond the walls of the faith community.

Reverend Richard Cathell and the Faith Community Nurses of Bellingham, Washington

Let's listen to Reverend Richard Cathell's story.

I assumed this position in 2009 after the parish nurse coordinator left to pursue other opportunities. I was approached by the hospital administration to take over the leadership of the parish nurse program. Initially, I was skeptical about taking on this responsibility; after all, I was a chaplain, not a nurse. But then I remembered that Granger Westberg, who had started parish nursing, was not a nurse, but a minister. I agreed to assume this leadership role only if the hospital agreed to allocate some funding for leadership. The hospital agreed to supply stipends for two parish nurses. I am budgeted at 20 percent of salary for my leadership role with faith community nurses.

I had observed that, typically, the parish nurse-coordinator felt a sense of isolation and loneliness in that position. They didn't quite fit into the hospital system and tended to feel like outsiders; likewise, one person couldn't keep up with the diversified demands. I addressed this issue through the creation of a leadership team of two faith community nurses. One, Jeanne Brotherton, RN, MEd, PN, serves as the parish nurse education coordinator, and Dotty Marston, RN, MN, is the outreach coordinator. These two nurses meet with me weekly and support each other.

In addition, I expanded the leadership team with three nurses who volunteer their services. Tisch Lynch, RN, MEd, and LeAna Osterman, RN, HMA, serve as administrative consultants, and Pamela Colyar oversees special projects. Also joining them in their weekly meetings are two anthropology students per quarter from Western Washington University, who assist with surveys, assessment tools, and community connectedness.

The first order of business was to decide what the nurse should be called—*parish nurse* or *faith community nurse*? The group decided on *faith community nurse* to be more inclusive and in line with the *Scope and Standards* statement formulated by HMA and accepted by the ANA. However, we made a decision to communicate to faith communities that the individual communities were free to call their nurse whatever was comfortable for them. Many continued with *parish nurse;* some chose to use *congregational nurse* or *church nurse*. A parish nurse by any other name is still a parish nurse!

In sixteen short months, the six of us—the two nurse-coordinators, along with the three additional volunteer nurses, and I—have done amazing things. We worked with the hospital library to have three large shelves set aside as a Health and Wellness section, with the entire bibliography listed on our website—books, DVDs. This provides a resource for faith community nurses. Access to the medical library is available twenty-four hours a day via their name badge bar code.

We decided that we needed a website. We already had a page on the hospital's website, which was under reconstruction, but we didn't have the freedom to modify our page to convey the message that we wanted to give those who viewed our web page. So we decided to independently create our own website, believing that a good website was key to a successful program. Our webmaster, Charles Nelson, PhD, is a retired archaeology professor who used to teach at the University of Nairobi. His sister, Sue Wright, is one of the local faith community nurses. Charles does more than the technical aspects of developing the site—he is able to ask questions of the team that help us to articulate our mission and what we want those who come to our site to know about us. That is, what do we want to communicate to our community at large? The result is that we have a wonderful website that can be accessed at www.health ministriesnetwork.net. We track the number of hits to the website and 22 percent are from outside the United States—from China, Russia, Australia, South Africa, India, Sri Lanka, and other countries.

Another project that we took on was to involve the FCN in discharge planning. Prior to discharge, the social workers at St. Joseph's Hospital ask patients if they are willing to meet an FCN pre-discharge and to be visited by the FCN after discharge. Once that permission is obtained and HIPAA requirements are met, the social workers can go to our website to find FCNs by city and congregation in order to match up the patient with a nearby FCN. The social worker gathers contact information through the website for an FCN to make a hospital pre-discharge patient visit. This is followed by at least one visit in the patient's home post-discharge followed by two to three telephone calls for follow-up. The FCN checks medications to make sure the patient has the correct ones and assesses the degree to which the patient is complying with the prescribed medication regimen, as well as diet issues and other aspects of the discharge plan. The FCN's approach is primarily geared to coaching the patient to follow the discharge instructions. This approach has decreased recidivism, or rehospitalization, by 30 percent, according to studies done by Eric Coleman, MD, of the University of Colorado Health Science Center.

We partnered with a company called Qualis, which is under contract to Medicare, to decrease rehospitalization costs among elderly patients. The Qualis program teaches nurses a coaching technique and the training is similar to that received by FCNs, except that there is no emphasis on meeting the spiritual needs of patients. Several of the FCNs have been trained by Qualis, and currently Qualis is interested in training its employees in the spiritual component of care.

I wanted to expand the role of FCNs and to create a health ministry network (HMN), so I brought together community organizations, congregations, FCNs, and six hospital departments to work collaboratively in providing coordinated services to the broader community. We focus on preventive health care, social justice, and spiritual nurture. Though this can be unwieldy, amazing things happen with all this energy and commitment to serve the community, providing huge networking opportunities—both collaborative and cooperative. Most FCNs traditionally focus on their own faith communities, but the HMN leadership team believes the role is broader than that and should include community neighbors within a geographical boundary, rather than limiting the services of an FCN to members within her congregation. Though there are various fears and resistances in making home visits to strangers, proper training and mentoring can help not only facilitate safe encounters, but also create an expanded neighborhood network.

Another issue that needed addressing was that many nurses interested in becoming FCNs found the length of the training (forty hours) too difficult to fit in with full-time jobs and families. As soon as the IPNRC came out with the new thirty-two-hour curriculum, the Bellingham, Washington, FCNs presented one of the first Basic Training courses in the Northwest. Still another issue was the cost of the training—which was about $400. One of the FCNs, Tisch Lynch, received an inheritance from her mother and she donated $2,000 to establish the Jean Billings Tischler Parish Nurse Educational Fund with the St. Luke's Foundation, a local community charity. This kind generosity was shared with the hospital foundation and others, who also made significant contributions. Thus, this year we were able to offer training for $100—we encourage each nurse to pay $50 and her congregation to pay $50. This has resulted in doubling the enrollment numbers.

Currently there are 102 FCNs, fifty-seven congregations, twenty community organizations, and six hospital departments. Sixteen months ago there were 69 parish nurses, forty-one congregations, with no community organizations and no hospital departments involved.

Another unique aspect of our program is that we allow nurses who are not affiliated with a faith community to become FCNs—so-called independent FCNs. The population in Bellingham is 85 percent unchurched—yet still spiritual. The same holds true for many communities, thus giving FCNs an opportunity to serve the community at large. For instance, a Buddhist FCN serves in an elder care lawyer's office; a Protestant FCN practices in an adult day care center. Though they are not functioning officially within a congregational setting, they can still provide wholistic care in community settings.

Like everything else in today's health care settings, there are many challenges that remain. But I believe that by working together as community leaders and organizations, cooperative networking brings out the best in everyone. We have nothing to fear from the future, unless we forget the way that God has led us in the past.

And how has God led us in the past? How is the development of FCN/PN reflective of God's leading? An example from scripture answers these questions. In Exodus 18:18–24 we hear how Moses, overwhelmed by the needs of the Israelites for counsel and judgment, was instructed by his father-in-law, Jethro, to establish a system of judges that could handle the minor problems of the Israelites, freeing up Moses to deal with the most important issues facing the fledgling nation. Moses needed a network of listeners, decision makers, and problem solvers so that he could fulfill the role that God intended for him

Among the tribes of the desert it was, and still is, customary for the sheikh of the tribe to sit in front of his tent for a short period each morning. During this period, various members of the tribe bring their disputes and grievances to him and he rules on these matters. Moses was trying to fill this role for the Israelites. The trouble was obvious to Jethro, Moses's father-in-law! Although this system was practical for the average desert tribe, it was completely impractical for a group the size of the Israelites. Moses had to hold court all day, every day, and the people who needed to see him were forced to stand around his tent for long periods, waiting for their turn to have their dispute adjudicated. Doubtless, Moses was aware that this was not the change to a smooth-running operation a leader likes to preside over, but his limited experience as a leader had not provided him with an alternative solution. Fortunately, his wise father-in-law, a leader among his own people, immediately suggested a practical solution. Under the new decentralized arrangement, the Israelites were divided into groups and subgroups, with leaders over groups of thousands and leaders over groups of hundreds and leaders over groups of fifty to one hundred or so, and leaders over groups of ten to fifty. The leader of each subgroup handled everyday complaints and disputes. The more difficult cases were still brought to Moses, but having these assistants freed him from the lesser matters that had been robbing him of time and energy.

FCNs also thrive on structure and organization, and their gifts and services can be used more effectively to serve not only those within their own faith communities but those beyond who are in need of the compassion and spiritual nurture that comes from the nurse's ministrations.

Faith community/parish nursing has come a long way. FCNs are recognized by the American Nurses Association; they are members of a professional membership organization of their own; they have a formal document detailing the scope and standards of practice of their profession as well as plans to recognize the expertise of parish nurses through credentialing; and they even debate about expanding the role of the parish nurse—all signs that this specialty has achieved professional status, recognition, and accountability.

These achievements, so valued by the secular health care system, are not necessarily the measure of quality within the sacred system of the church. Sometimes, what the secular system promotes is clearly at odds with the values of ministry, service, compassion, love of God and neighbor, and the importance of community—all upheld by the church. Today there are nurses who are quietly expressing fears about this movement toward standardization, credentialing, and third-party reimbursement. Their voices express concern that parish nursing could become so secularized as to be no different from the disillusioning model of nursing that currently prevails in the health care system. Their voices express a belief that the specialty is first and foremost a response to God's call and as such is primarily accountable to God and God's church.

These contrasting views produce tension within the parish nurse movement. Currently, the tension is felt as a gentle undercurrent; over time the tension may pull at the very fabric of parish nursing. Already there are parish nurses employed by hospital systems who are struggling to straddle the divide between the values and priorities of the sacred church system and the secular health care system. This tension will only be effectively dealt with if it is openly confronted with continuing dialogue between the church and the health care system.

We also predict that as the secular health care system recognizes the value of the parish nurse to increase the market share and the profitability of the system, there will be a sharper delineation within the practice arena between parish nursing as a ministry with allegiance to God and congregation and parish nursing as a department of a health care system. We also predict that, in response to this delineation, both Christian and non-Christian faith traditions will increase their involvement and ownership in parish nursing as part of wholistic health ministries, thus ensuring their "place at the table" in dialogues with health care systems regarding values and mission.

Most parish nurses practicing today serve in unpaid positions, giving freely of their time because of the strength of their call and commitment to this ministry. We believe that this needs to change, and, indeed, will change. Parish nurses need to be paid. Whether the nurse's salary comes from the church, the health care system, or a partnership between the church and the health care system, the source of her salary is not nearly as important as the fact that she is paid. We tend to value things and services that cost us something and when something is free we tend to dismiss it as less valuable. A salary is a concrete sign that the nurse's services are not only important and appreciated, but that the parish nurse's role is a credible and respected one within the church. Again, as churches and health care systems recognize the contributions made by parish nurses, there will be greater willingness to budget for salaries.

Years ago, Reverend Granger Westberg wished for a thousand churches, each with a parish nurse program. His wish came true. We are so convinced of the importance of parish nurses that we dare to dream even bigger than Reverend Westberg did. We dream of a time when there will be a paid parish nurse in every congregation!

Education

Many parish nurses who shared their stories reported taking a preparation course that had been endorsed by the International Parish Nurse Resource Center (IPNRC) and offered at an institution approved by the same group. The pioneering efforts of the IPNRC are to be applauded. This organization created a solid foundation for the development of parish nursing as a specialty. The IPNRC's emphasis on standardization has served parish nursing well in launching and expanding the specialty as well as in garnering professional recognition for FCNs. However, there are signs that the educational preparation of parish nurses will also change as the specialty moves forward.

We predict that the changes will fall into the following four categories. First, there will be greater curricular development related to parish nursing within university-based schools of nursing, with the faculty of these schools taking ownership of the objectives, content, and flow of the courses based on the *Scope and Standards of Practice*. This change is in line with the traditional role of the faculty to take responsibility for curricular development. There will be clinical experiences designed for the undergraduate as well as the graduate student in nursing. Currently, an increasing number of undergraduate nursing students are assigned to work alongside FCNs as part of a practicum.[7]

Second, there will be an increasing number of graduate programs in parish nursing with an emphasis on research into the efficacy of the parish nurse role and with recognition that the advanced practice nurse has a place within a congregational health ministry.[8] Third, FCN/parish nurse preparation courses, provided by Christian-based organizations, will add spiritual content to the standardized IPNRC curriculum to maintain the original Christian identity of parish nursing. This is already happening, not only within the FCN/parish nurse preparation courses across the country, but in the efforts of individual FCNs to take additional courses in seminaries to better prepare themselves to respond to the spiritual needs of those they serve.[9]

A review of nursing literature reveals a growing body of research concerning parish nursing. The research points to the "youth" of the movement in that the primary focus of research efforts is on "what exists" within the field. For instance, there are studies that examine the meaning and experience of parish nursing,[10] a comparison of the roles of the rural versus the urban parish nurse,[11] an exploration of congregants' perceptions of the distinctive aspects of nursing practice within a congregation,[12] and descriptions of parish nursing practice using the Nursing Minimum Data Set.[13]

A 2008 study by McGinnis and Zoske[14] focused on the importance of the FCN in prevention and management of chronic disease—especially among the elderly. Increasingly, FCNs are reaching into the neighborhoods surrounding their faith communities and offering services to those who tend to fall through the cracks of the health care system—the poor, those who are homeless, and immigrant populations. A research study conducted by Mendelson et al. (2008)[15] reported significant differences in glycemic control, macrosomia, and days of maternal and/or neonatal hospitalization between the groups of Mexican American women with gestational diabetes who received the parish nurse intervention, compared to the group who received care as usual. Other areas of potential study include evaluating the effectiveness of the teaching role of the FCN. Does health education make a difference beyond anecdotal reports? Do congregants make behavior changes based on what the nurse has taught? Health-related screenings, such as blood pressure and cholesterol screenings, are also reported as important interventions by parish nurses. Do these parish nurse interventions lead to lifestyle changes among congregants? Certainly, the research reported by Rydholm et al. (2007) and Brown et al. (2009) provides evidence that the efforts of FCNs to educate result in decreased health care costs. We need more of these well-designed studies.

Another area for research is the relationship between faith and health. For instance, a common theme among the nurses who shared their stories with us was the effectiveness of prayer and the importance of visiting congregants either in the hospital, in a nursing home, or in the congregant's own home. An appropriate demonstration project for parish nursing might be first to examine the effectiveness of prayer. Does prayer correlate with decreased anxiety or depression, increased hope, and/or increased acceptance of and peace in approaching death? Another study might compare the effect of home or hospital visits with and without prayer. The role of the parish nurse offers countless opportunities to study the relationship between faith and various aspects of health as well as to examine the effectiveness of specific faith-based interventions, such as prayer, participation in worship service, and receiving communion. The territory is ripe for research into faith community/parish nursing, and the studies have only just begun.

We anticipate a future where the concept of faith community nursing will not only exist within individual faith communities but increasingly will reach into the surrounding communities to provide spiritual sustenance, health education, preventive interventions, and advocacy for those who may not belong to a specific faith community, but are still in need.

We conclude this book with one last story by Laura Rydholm,[16] who, along with others who share her vision of faith community/ parish nursing, conducted and published the first outcome studies on the effectiveness of this God-given and -ordained specialty. Laura's story in many ways is a summation of this book. She talks about the call, the response to the call, the sacredness of relationships, and the interventions and the outcomes.

I think a lot of us were parish nurses before they ever gave it a title, especially in ultrarural settings. The folks we shared communion with would ask for advice about symptoms as a way of making conversation: It was part of the morning ritual. Oftentimes, over coffee in the basement of the church, between discussions about the weather and the price of lumber, members would mention the ailments of the week. After sharing how much rain had fallen on their crops the day before, they might compare cholesterol levels, and successes or failures with herbal remedies. Once in a while, someone would call because they didn't want to bother 911, but most of the important work involved listening and remembering what was said. My growing understanding of the people I was serving became my expertise. Knowing their histories, vulnerabilities, and coping patterns helped me become the advocate they needed in times of crisis. It changes a person when people learn to trust you with their secrets and well-being. It makes you more humble, more vulnerable, less concerned about the lab values and more concerned about matters of the heart.

Ultrarural nurses in small congregations aren't hired—they simply show up, and eventually become recognized for their talents in advocacy. Lu Vitalis and Annette Langdon describe the process of evolving into the role as "a calling and a falling." It is important to recognize that nurses are not the only ones this happens to. Ideally, all of us find a way to offer our unique gifts to community in a way that is life-sustaining. Gary Gunderson put it well when he said that health ministry is something that everyone in the congregation is doing 24/7. Still, it is worth noting that the presence of guardians, such as parish nurses, is one of the solutions to the current health care crisis. Persuading people to access care before their deteriorating conditions end in permanent disabilities is a valuable art.

Granger Westberg can be credited with telling the world that this resource should be leveraged, but nurses have been doing the work of supporting the downtrodden informally for centuries, and good people will undoubtedly continue to serve where they are needed, An opportunity to troubleshoot the health care crisis is being lost in the sense that intentionality diminishes wherever the role remains unfunded, but it's no surprise that the ability to keep people out of the system is undervalued by formal providers.

My interest in capturing outcomes was kindled in 1990. Parish nurses were emerging in Iowa in droves at the time, under the remarkable leadership of Jan Striepe. I remember being cut to the quick when Jan was dismayed that we weren't making an impact on paper. Jan was gathering minimal parish nurse notes for the NW Iowa Agency on Aging under a Kellogg Project at the time, because none of us were in it for the charting opportunity. I was bothered by the comment because I had just persuaded yet another elder to seek care before looming intubation became necessary. I remember how strongly I felt that this story needed to be heard. The man who couldn't breathe had sought me out because he didn't know where else to turn. When he found me, he casually asked, in a breathless manner, if I would check his blood pressure. I asked him why he hadn't gone to the physician directly. In halting phrases he denied being short of breath, but confessed that he didn't want to admit that his efforts to stop smoking had failed. Upon being redirected to a new physician "who would understand," surprisingly he was sent home with four new prescriptions. Not surprisingly, he rapidly retained fluids in response to the new high doses of steroids. Accordingly, he threatened to stop all medications because they were making him fat. I remember how he reluctantly consented to let me help him bother the doctor for diuretics and how happy he was to report the loss of fifteen pounds the next day after the needed prescription was obtained. Even more reluctantly, he consented to have his potassium checked and replenished the day after that. I recall thinking that, since this was a typical inpatient scenario for someone with COPD in the 1980s, the government owed me a thank-you note for managing it informally. I imagine many people feel this way from time to time. I knew I couldn't be the only one having this experience.

My opportunity to capture, collate, and communicate outcomes came when I was hired by Immanuel St. Joseph's to launch parish nurse programs in South Central Minnesota. Under a federal grant, we acquired more than two thousand stories using the DIARY format (a variation of Susan Lampe's FOCUS charting system). The stories were distilled. Concerns, interventions, and outcomes were summarized and cost savings resulting from interventions were demonstrated. Our shared experience was then published in *Holistic Nursing Practice*, and we did get a thank-you note from the Administration on Aging in Washington, D.C.

Subsequently, with the invaluable help of people like Wanda Alexander, the study was replicated with support from the state of Minnesota and the Medica Foundation, a predominant third-party payer. This time the nurses were based in metropolitan congregations, and many of them were functioning in paid roles. Again the cost-saving aspect of the role was evident. More importantly, the interventions reported by these nurses echoed the rural stories. Recently, Canadian nurses have reported similar experiences in a nationally funded project comparing interventions of nurses in churches with those of nurses in community centers and nurses in retirement village settings. None of this journey was planned, of course. It all just fell together over time. It will be interesting to see what door opens next.

As we conclude this book about the stories of parish nurses and parish nursing, we hope that you have enjoyed accompanying us on this journey. The story of parish nursing is a story of call, response, journey, and faith. We began by listening to nurses describe their call to ministry. Sometimes the call was strong and clear; at other times it was vague but persistent. Likewise the response was sometimes immediate and wholehearted; at other times it was delayed and initially tentative. All responses were acts of faith.

We listened to the nurses' words as they described the details of the journey—the highs and lows, the joys and sorrows. We heard them describe how God has led them not just to ministry within their own congregations but to ministry beyond the church to surrounding communities of need. We listened as they described the importance of health education, of listening, of being present to others and offering the love of God to those in need.

We listened as they talked about their preparation for the journey. We listened as they described their sources of support and their increasing efforts to organize and to standardize their practice through local and state networks and at the national and international levels through the efforts of the International Parish Nurse Resource Center (IPNRC), accessible via www.parishnurses.org. The global reach of the IPNRC allows parish nurses to provide education, written resources, and loving guidance—as well as prayer support—to nurses like Shazhad Gill, who courageously serves his church community in Pakistan; to Dr. Emmerentia du Plessis, who is developing her ministry in South Africa; and to other nurses who are scattered around the world and responding to the same call from a loving God to bring care to those in need.

One theme consistently present throughout the stories of parish nurses is that this ministry is ordained by God. An acceptance of this as truth leads us to believe that God will continue to guide and shape this clinical practice. How it will occur is something about which we can only speculate. There is an old saying: "Man plans and God smiles." And so as we bring closure to this book with our predictions as well as our hopes for parish nurses and parish nursing, we can take comfort in the belief that Someone indeed may be smiling.

Notes

Introduction

1. Ferngren, G. B. (1992). Early Christianity as a religion of healing. *Bulletin of the History of Medicine*, 66, 13–14.

2. Koenig, H. G., McCullough, M. E., & Larson, D. B. (2001). *Handbook of religion and health*. New York: Oxford University Press, 29.

3. Carson, V. B. (1989). *Spiritual dimensions of nursing practice*. Philadelphia: W. B. Saunders, 55–56.

4. McNamara, K. (2000, Spring/Summer). Remembered forever. *Perspectives in Faith Community/Parish Nursing Practice*, 12. This is a tribute to Reverend Westberg written by his granddaughter. He died on February 16, 1999.

5. American Nurses Association. (2005). *Faith community nursing: Scope and standards of practice*. Washington, D.C.: American Nurses Association Publishing.

Chapter 1

1. K. Barker (Ed.). (1985). *The NIV study bible*. Grand Rapids, Mich.: Zondervan Publishing House, 379–80.

2. "The Summons," text by J. L. Bell, ©1987. GIA Publications, Inc.

Chapter 2

1. Westberg, G. (1987). *The parish nurse: How to start a parish nurse program in your church*. Park Ridge, Ill.: Parish Nurse Resource Center, 8–9.

2. Holstrom, S. (1999). Perspectives on a suburban practice. In A. Solari-Twadell and M. A. McDermott (Eds.), *Parish nursing: Promoting whole person health within faith communities* (69–73). Thousand Oaks, Calif.: Sage Publications; Clark, M. B., & Olson, J. K. (2000). *Nursing within a faith community: Promoting health in times of transition*. Thousand Oaks, Calif.: Sage Publications, 141–54.

3. Carson, V. B., & Koenig, H. G. (2002). *Spiritual caregiving: Healthcare as a ministry*. Philadelphia: Templeton Foundation Press.

4. Medvene, L., et al. (2003). Promoting signing of advance directives in faith communities. *Journal of General Internal Medicine*, 18(11), 914–20.

5. Dr. Judy Shelly, editor of the *Journal of Christian Nursing*, author of many publications, and parish nurse at St. Luke's Lutheran Church in Obelisk, Pennsylvania.

6. Swinney, J., Anson-Wonka, C., Maki, E., & Corneau, J. (2001, January–February). Community assessment: A church community and the parish nurse, *Public Health Nursing* 18(1), 40–44.

7. R. S. Young, from *Parish Nursing Report* (February 2001), for New Virginia United Methodist Church in Hermitage, Pennsylvania. Also from Kelly Preston's story of her role as congregational health program coordinator of Baptist Health System in Alabama. Also, T. Pruski (2000, August 10). Our congregations: Where physical and spiritual health can prevail. *The Catholic Standard*, a publication of the Archdiocese of Washington, D.C. Pruski is health and wellness coordinator of Wellness Works Catholic Charities of Montgomery County. Also from Marianne Parker's story: Marianne shared the results of a survey conducted by St. Joseph's Hospital Congregational Health Program and summarized over four thousand health promotion contacts and two thousand hours of volunteer time donated to the twenty-nine churches active in the program, the five churches that are forming a congregational health ministry, and the fifteen churches that are interested in forming a congregational ministry.

8. Buijs, R., & Olson, J. (2001). Parish nurses influencing determinants of health. *Journal of Community Health Nursing*, 18(1), 13–23.

9. *Fiscal Year 2010 in Brief.* (2010). U.S. Department of Health & Human Services Fiscal Year 2010 Budget in Brief—Medicare. Retrieved from http://www.hhs.gov?asrt/ob/docbudget/2010budgetinbriefl.html.

10. Parker, M. (2000, Summer). Mobilizing volunteers for service. *Healing Hearts and Hands*, 4(3), 1. This is a publication edited by Marianne Parker, congregational health ministry coordinator for St. Joseph's Hospital Health Center in Syracuse, New York. The publication is an example of the teaching/communication resources developed by parish nurses. In this issue, Marianne discusses how to mobilize volunteers, examines the sources of tension and provides wholistic suggestions to deal with tension, provides a calendar of upcoming community events, announces upcoming seminars and networking opportunities for parish nurses, shares stories of parish nurses, publishes prayer requests, inserts articles highlighting vision research as well as vision for ministry—both requiring periodic examination, and offers suggestions for parish nurses to support biblical parenting.

11. Oman, D., Thoresen, C., & McMahon, K. (1999). Volunteerism and

mortality among the community-dwelling elderly. *Journal of Health Psychology*, 4(3), 301–16; Freedman, M. (1999). *Prime time: How baby boomers will revolutionize retirement and transform America.* New York: Public Affairs; Koenig, H. G. (2002). *Purpose and power in retirement.* Philadelphia: Templeton Foundation Press.

12. Parker, Mobilizing volunteers for service.

13. Gaul, C. (2001, June 21). If you ask them, they will come. *The Catholic Review*, 67(10), 1, 3.

14. Parker, Mobilizing volunteers for service.

15. Eileen Altenhofer was parish nurse coordinator at Normandy Park Congregational Church in Seattle, Washington. In June 1999, Eileen stepped down from the position of parish nurse coordinator but continues to support the health ministry in her church as a parish care committee resource member. Joan Wieringa shared the position of parish nurse coordinator with Eileen and now has continued in the role of coordinator, a role that became a paid position in January 1999.

16. Buijs & Olson, Parish nurses influencing determinants of health.

17. Parker, Mobilizing volunteers for service.

Chapter 3

1. Carson, V. B. (2000). *Mental health nursing: The nurse-patient journey*, 2nd ed. Philadelphia: W. B. Saunders & Company, 3.

Chapter 4

1. (2001). *The soul Bible.* Nashville: Thomas Nelson Publishers, 1250.

2. Rydholm, L., et al. (2008). Care of community-dwelling older adults by faith community nurses. *Journal of Gerontological Nursing*, 34(4); Rydholm, L. (1995). *Project 309-95: Summary of parish nurse visits for MN region nine area agency on aging.* Mankato, Minn.; Rydholm, L. (1997). *Outcome-based charting: Benefits of DIARY narrative vs. charting-by-exception approaches to storytelling.* Westberg Symposium XI papers. (Park Ridge, Ill.: International Parish Nurse Resource Center); Rydholm, L. (1997). Patient-focused care in parish nursing. *Holistic Nursing Practice*, 11, 47–60.

3. Wanda Alexander, parish nurse and community health supervisor for Hennepin County Human Services and Public Health Department (HSPHD) and the Faith Community Network, decided to conduct a survey to determine who practiced as FCNs, in what congregations, and the nature of their work in those congregations. Two faculty members from the University of Minnesota School of Nursing contracted to conduct the research in collaboration with HSPHD. The survey was developed in collaboration with

the latter and the Faith Community Nurse Network. It was sent to a list of FCNs practicing in the thirteen-county metropolitan areas of the Twin Cities by HSPHD staff. FCNs were reimbursed for their time by the Faith Community Nurse Network when the survey was returned. Data were coded by the research staff at the School of Nursing. Respondent confidentiality was assured. This report included the responses of 144 currently practicing FCNs. There were 237 surveys mailed and 176 returned. Of those returned, 20 were former FCNs and 12 were incomplete or came from individuals who were not FCNs. The responses from former FCNs were not included in the summary. The response rate for the entire survey was 74 percent and for the 144 currently practicing FCNs 61 percent.

4. The video that Kristine refers to presents the stories of four women who have been victims of domestic violence. Two of the women are from the Protestant tradition, one is a Roman Catholic, and the other is Jewish. After these women present their stories, clergy from each faith tradition respond. The video is available from the Center for Prevention of Sexual and Domestic Violence in Seattle, Washington.

5. Cooney, R. (1994). "Jerusalem, My Destiny." In R. J. Batastini and M. A. Cymbala (Eds.). *Gather* (2nd ed). Chicago: GIA Publications, Inc.

Chapter 5

1. Quindlen, A. (2000). *A short guide to a happy life.* New York: Random House.

2. Albom, M. (1997). *Tuesdays with Morrie.* New York: Doubleday.

3. McCormick, P. (2001). Pass it on. *U.S. Catholic,* 66(8), 46–48.

4. Anonymous. (1989, Winter). Parish nursing's pioneer: A JCN interview with Granger Westberg. *Journal of Community Nursing,* 6(1), 26–29.

5. Solari-Twadell, P. A., & McDermott, M. A. (1999). *Parish nursing: Promoting whole person health within faith communities.* Thousand Oaks, Calif.: Sage Press, 269–75.

6. See http://www.hmassoc.org/assets/.../norma%20w-d%20award%20 2003.pdf.

7. Edman, E. (2009). *Out of the Clinic and into the Church. The Covenant Companion.* Retrieved from http://www.covchurch.org/uploads/G6/Jr/G6Jru Tbe3vutrRrGywMs4w/Out-of-the-Clinic.pdf.

8. Northwest Parish Nurse Ministries. (2010). *History of northwest parish nursing.* Portland, Ore.: Northwest Parish Nurse Ministries.

Chapter 6

1. (1994). *The NIV quiet time Bible.* Downers Grove, Ill.: InterVarsity Press.

2. Shelly, J. A., & Miller, A. B. (1999). *Called to care: A Christian theology of nursing.* Downers Grove: Ill.: InterVarsity Press.

3. Anonymous. (1989, Winter). Parish nursing's pioneer: A JCN interview with Granger Westberg. *Journal of Community Nursing,* 6(1), 26–29.

4. Westberg, G. (1987). *The parish nurse: How to start a parish nurse program in your church.* Park Ridge, Ill.: Parish Nurse Resource Center, 8–9.

5. Health Ministries Association, Inc., & American Nurses Association. (2005). *Scope and standards of faith community nursing practice.* Washington, D.C.: American Nurses Association Publishing.

6. Perkin, K. (2007). Parish nursing and hospitals. *Health Progress,* 88(1), 44–47.

7. Remsen, J. (2001, August 5). A pioneering Jewish "congregational" nurse offers holistic care: Ministering to the body and soul. *Philadelphia Inquirer.*

8. Koenig, H., & Larson, D. (2004). *Faith in the future: Healthcare, aging, and the role of religion.* Philadelphia: Templeton Foundation Press.

9. Smith, S. D. (2003). *Parish nursing: A handbook for the new millennium.* Binghamton, N.Y.: Haworth Press.

10. Rosemarie Matheus, director of the Parish Nurse Preparation Institute at Marquette University College of Nursing, shared her insights regarding parish nursing in a taped interview that she graciously made for the first edition of this book in spring 2001.

11. Striepe, J. M., & King, J. M. (1993, Winter). Basics of beginning a parish nurse program. *Journal of Christian Nursing,* 10(1), 14–17; Maddox, M. (2001, Summer). Circle of Christian Caring: A model for nursing practice. *Journal of Christian Nursing,* 11–13.

12. Miller, L. W. (1997). Nursing through the lens of faith: A conceptual model. *Journal of Christian Nursing,* 14(1), 17–20.

13. Koenig, H., & Larson, D. *Faith in the future.*

14. O'Brien, M. E. (2010). *Servant leadership in nursing: Spirituality and practice in contemporary health care.* Sudbury, Mass.: Jones and Bartlett Publishers.

15. Robert K. Greenleaf's 1970 essay, titled "Servant Leadership," retrieved from Greenleaf Center for Servant Leadership, http://www.greenleaf.org.

16. Smith, S. (2003). *Parish nursing: A handbook for the new millennium.* Binghamton, N.Y.: Haworth Press.

Chapter 7

1. Striepe, J. M., & King, J. M. (1993). Basics for beginning a faith community/parish nurse program. *Journal of Christian Nursing*, 10(1), 17.

2. Westberg, G. (1990). *The parish nurse*. Minneapolis: Augsburg Fortress Press.

Chapter 8

1. American Nurses Association. (2005). *Faith community nursing: Scope and standards of practice*. Washington, D.C.: American Nurses Association Publishing.

2. Information on levels of faith community nursing preparation from IPNRC available at http://www.parishnurse.org/Home.

3. Brown, I., et al. (2009). Faith community nursing demonstrates good stewardship of community benefit dollars through cost savings and cost avoidance. *Community Health*, 32(4), 333.

4. Rydholm, L., et al. Care of community-dwelling older adults by faith community nurses. *Journal of Gerontological Nursing*, 34(4), 2008.

5. Rydholm, L. (1997). Patient-focused care in parish nursing. *Holistic Nursing Practice*, 11, 47–60.

6. Brown, I., et al. Faith community nursing demonstrates good stewardship of community benefit dollars through cost savings and cost avoidance.

7. Kotecki, C. N. (2002). Community-based strategies: Incorporating faith-based partnerships into the curriculum. *Nurse Educator*, 27(1), 13–15.

8. Magilvy, J. K., & Brown, N. J. (1997). Parish nursing: Advanced practice nursing. Model for healthier communities. *Advanced Practice Nursing Quarterly*, 2(4), 67–72.

9. Brudenell, I. (2003). Parish nursing: Nurturing body, mind, spirit, and community. *Public Health Nursing*, 20(2), 85–94.

10. Chase-Zolke, M. (1999). The meaning and experience of health ministry within the culture of a congregation with a parish nurse. *Journal of Transcultural Nursing*, 10(1), 46–55.

11. Chase-Zolke, M., & Striepe, J. (1999). A comparison of urban versus rural experiences of nurses volunteering to promote health in churches. *Public Health Nursing*, 16(4), 270–79.

12. Chase-Zolken, M., & Gruca, J. (2000). Client's perceptions of distinctive aspects in nursing care within a congregational setting. *Journal of Community Health Nursing*, 17(3), 171–83.

13. Coenen, A., et al. (1999). Describing parish nurse practice using the Nursing Minimum Data Set. *Public Health Nursing*, 16(6), 412–16.

17. McGinnis, S. L., & Zoske, F. M. (2008). The emerging role of faith community nurse in prevention and management of chronic disease. *Policy, Politics & Nursing Practice*, 9(3), 173–80.

15. Mendelson, S. G., et al. (2008). A community-based parish nurse intervention program for Mexican American women with gestational diabetes. *Journal of Gynecologic and Neonatal Nursing*, 37(4), 415–25.

16. Rydholm, L., & Thornquist, L. (2005). Supporting seniors across systems: Effectiveness of parish nurse interventions. Metropolitan Area Agency on Aging research study, sponsored by Minnesota Department of Human Services with in-kind contributions from Hennepin County; Rydholm, L., et al. Care of community-dwelling older adults by faith community nurses; Rydholm, L. (1995). *Project 309-95: Summary of parish nurse visits for MN region nine area agency on aging*. Mankato, Minn.; Rydholm, L. (1997). *Outcome-based charting: Benefits of DIARY narrative vs. charting-by-exception approaches to storytelling*. Westberg Symposium XI papers. Park Ridge, Ill.: International Parish Nurse Resource Center; Rydholm, L. (1997). Patient-focused care in parish nursing. *Holistic Nursing Practice*, 11, 47–60.

Index

Index

Index

Index

Index